Bobbi Brown
LIVING BEAUTY

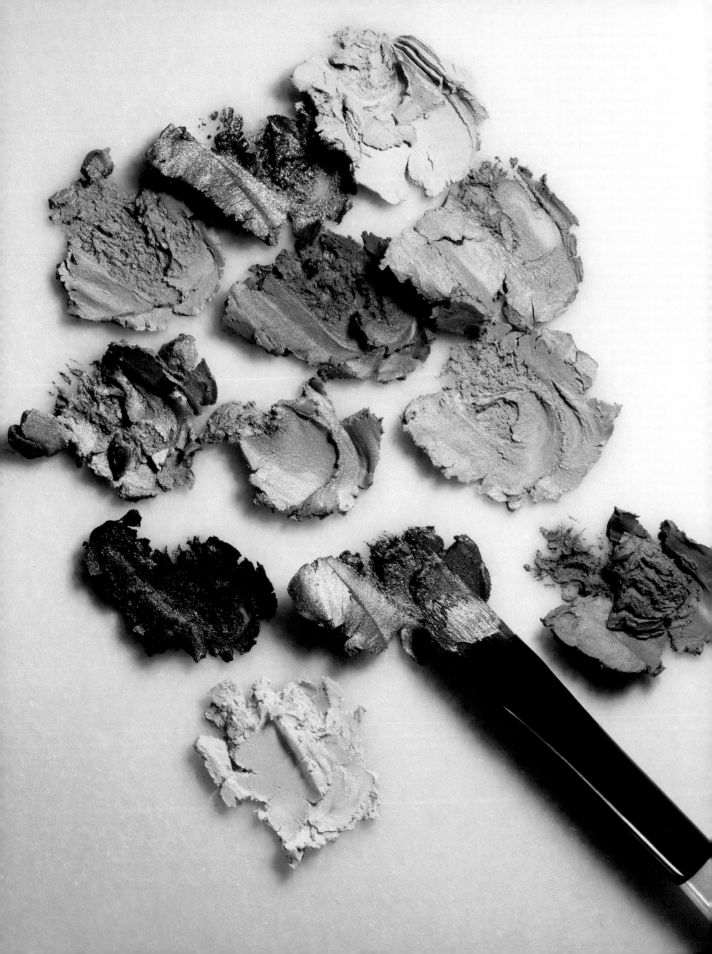

Bobbi Brown

LIVING BEAUTY

BOBBI BROWN WITH
MARIE CLARE KATIGBAK-SILLICK
PHOTOGRAPHS BY HENRY LEUTWYLER

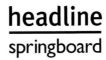

headline
springboard

First published in 2007 by
Springboard Press
An imprint of Warner Books, Inc
A division of Hachette Book Group USA

First published in Great Britain in 2007 by
Headline Springboard
An imprint of HEADLINE PUBLISHING GROUP

First published in paperback in Great Britain in 2010 by
Headline Springboard

1

Cataloguing in Publication Data is available from the British Library

ISBN 978 0 7553 1630 4

Printed and bound in the UK by the Butler Tanner and Dennis, Frome

Designed by Ruba Abu-Nimah, Kevin Ley and Tyler Askew
Photography by Henry Leutwyler
Except photograph on page 10: Stephen Danelian/Corbis Outline
Photograph on page 14: Matthias Clamer/Corbis Outline
Photograph on page 193: Kelly Klein

Headline's policy is to use papers that are natural, renewable and
recyclable products and made from wood grown in sustainable
forests. The logging and manufacturing processes are expected to
conform to the environmental regulations of the country of origin.

HEADLINE PUBLISHING GROUP
An Hachette UK Company
338 Euston Road
London NW1 3BH

www.headline.co.uk
www.hachette.co.uk

Style Note:
'Rx' denotes a remedy or
solution to a problem

As always, to the lights of my life—my boys.
Steven, my rock and my soul.
Dylan, Dakota, and Duke, my heart.

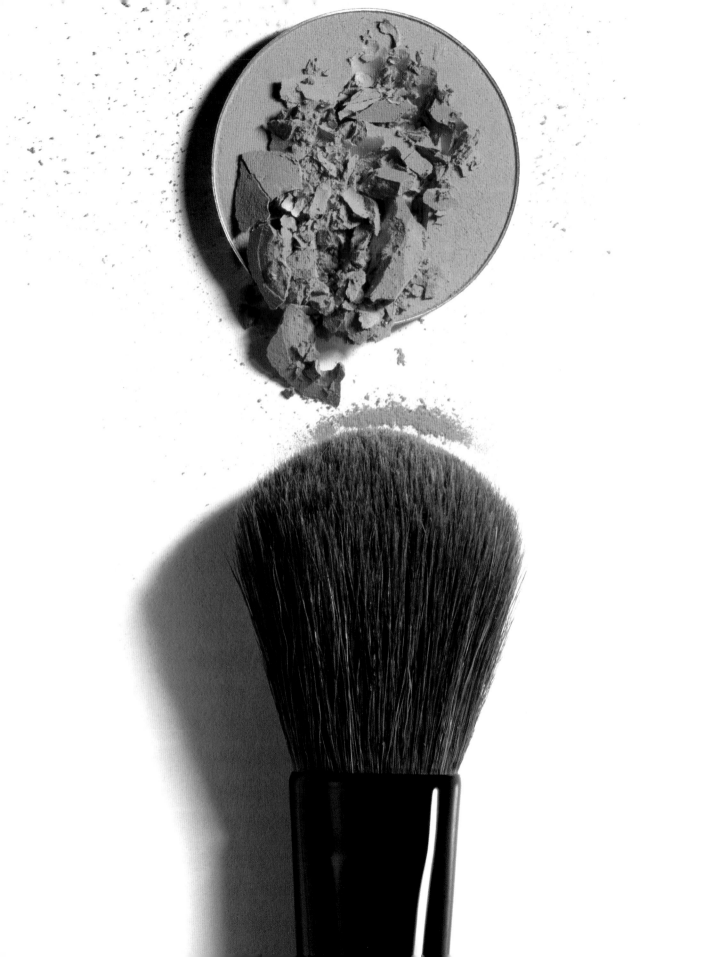

Contents

Foreword

By Debra Winger, New York, 2006

The prospect of writing about a woman "aging gracefully" has always given me pause. The term itself sounds as if one is lingering on each landing of a descending staircase, waving elegantly. The descent is what I do not like.

Aging, I feel, is more of an ascension; I like that it is an "ing" word. It denotes a process that is alive and happening, growing up and getting closer. Now, we all know what "closer" may mean, but I think of it as moving toward the essential: what was there in the beginning and will be there in the end. We spend a lot of time in between trying to mask our age, hide it, reshape it, but it usually looks just that way . . . an altered state.

I have tried in the last decade to abstain from value judgments of those who choose plastic surgery. I don't know enough about it to even remark. Sometimes the results are startling to the untrained eye, but many times I'm sure I don't notice what has been done. For me, though, I am actually *interested* in the process of aging as an unfolding of some mystery. When I was little, someone told me that when you age, you turn into the person you were all your life. My grandmother, although possessing beautiful skin, had a sort of permanent grimace that she called her smile. It did things to her face that said a lot. My mother, whom I didn't get to see age past seventy, had a twinkle in her eye that stole your attention immediately.

Each time I travel to another country and encounter another culture, when I return I am struck by the degree to which American culture is led by the media and not the lives and inherent beauty of its general population. This is not to say that everyone subscribes to this view, but it is safe to say that the popular culture has no room for real wrinkles. We are the specialists in no lines, no map, no history, and this includes the history of many other lands. My favorite state of mind is when I am not made to think about myself from the outside in. The fact is, this is a fool's errand. Through a series of events early in my life, I found that the message I got about "vision" is that you will never truly know what you look like to others, because it is your consciousness and your critical eye that are looking in the mirror. It is simply a measure of one's own compassion for oneself, which we all know is the first step to compassion for others.

It seems to me that the challenge is to be the embodiment of whatever is happening in your life at the moment. Sad faces can be extraordinarily moving and beautiful. Happiness is a message, not a look. Making it more difficult, the movie industry in the

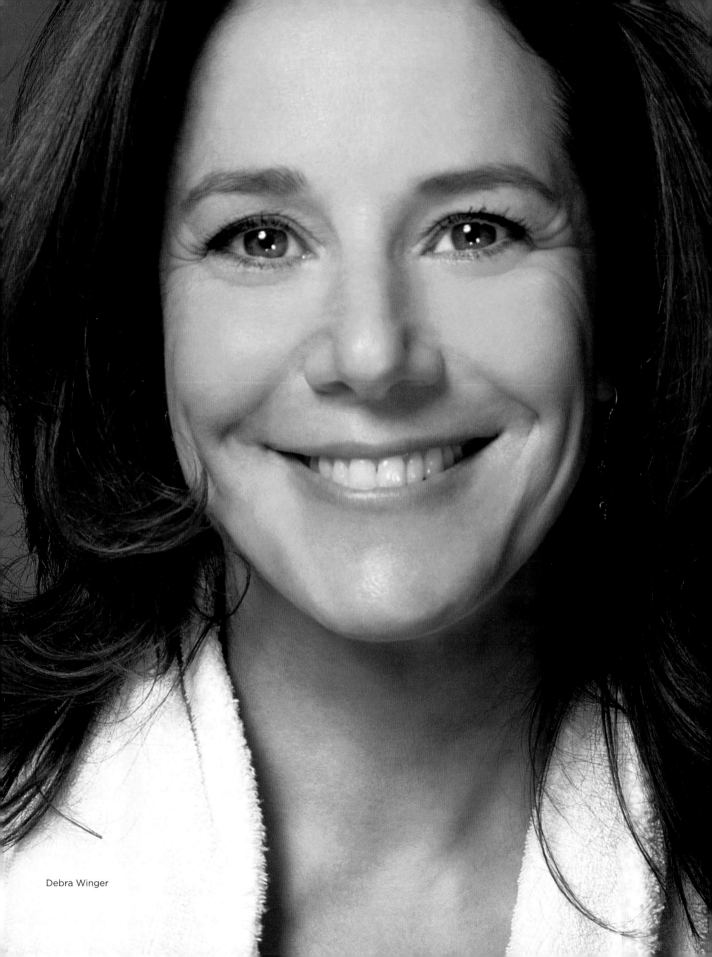

Debra Winger

United States promotes a lineless, motionless look for women of all ages that is, ironically, so nonthreatening that it is scary. But not "scary" in the way we want in the movies. Not in a way that would wake us up, kick us in the butt, and say, "Hey! Get on with it!"

The knowledge that Bobbi has shared begs the question of how palpable can beauty, enhanced or not, be without acceptance of oneself at every stage of life. I am interested in this question. I also applaud those who hold up different approaches to beauty. It is a big world and there is room for us all. A deeper understanding can only lead to a greater appreciation. The effects of our actions are written on our faces. Why not tell countless stories in many languages?

Introduction
The Living Beauty Philosophy

There's a certain amount of peace that comes with getting older. I realize this as I am entering my fifties (yikes!). After so many years of aspiring to unattainable ideals, I have finally learned to let go and relax. "Letting go" doesn't mean that I've stopped caring about my face, my hair, or my body. I still care, but I am more realistic about my expectations of myself. I am (finally) comfortable in my skin—and it is such a relief. Now my energy is focused on creating a new ideal, a new reality, and a new aspiration for myself—and that is the essence of *Living Beauty*.

I don't know why it's not OK to age. I think that a face without lines and planes is an expressionless face—it's a face that lacks warmth and confidence. That's why I'm dismayed at the number of women today who are altering their faces in an attempt to look younger. Visits to the plastic surgeon have become as commonplace as visits to the hair salon. I have to admit that there are some women who get nipped and tucked and actually look great. But I see many more who have been pulled so tight that they look completely artificial, and others who are so plumped up and frozen that they just look odd. There's a very fine line between plastic surgery that looks good and plastic surgery that looks plain awful. When you go under the knife there's no guarantee of the results—and no turning back.

Of course it's very easy to feel bad. Open any magazine and you're inundated by pictures of seemingly flawless girls who are barely twenty years old (and in some instances, as young as fourteen). Models older than thirty are a rarity. Television shows set in Los Angeles and New York glorify the lives of twenty-something characters. My advice? Don't compare yourself to these images of youthful perfection—you'll always lose. It's human nature to compare, but at least do it in a realistic way, with women close to your age.

I know a woman in her forties who's an average beauty, but who carries herself with above-average confidence. I ran into her once during fashion week and started complaining about how hard it was for me to be in a business surrounded by teenage models. She laughed and told me that I was in the wrong industry. As a successful attorney for a teamsters' union, she was surrounded by teamsters who thought she was "hot." She felt great about herself. There's another woman I know who's in her mid-sixties, but who says she still feels like a kid. She works as a music therapist at a senior citizens' home and is a few decades younger than many of the residents, who tell her she is stunning. So you see, beauty and aging are all relative.

Too many women of my generation feel bad about the fact that they're no longer young. These women have a laundry list of things they don't like about themselves—wrinkles, baggy eyelids, a too-small upper lip...I could go on for days. These women are so caught up in the negative that they don't have any energy left to focus on the positive.

I believe there needs to be a fundamental change in the way we think about beauty. We can either fall into this cycle of self-loathing, or we can empower ourselves with the knowledge to deal with the things that make us unhappy. I want to get rid of the stigma that surrounds aging. Aging (or getting older) should be seen as a process through which a woman can gain more vitality, strength, wisdom, and a new sense of her beauty. It really is an evolution. Today, there are many ways for women to be their best at any age. With knowledge, a strategy, and many lifestyle changes, women can feel better at forty, fifty, and sixty than they did ten, even twenty years ago.

No matter what your age, it's never too late to make a commitment to yourself. If you're feeling overwhelmed, I don't blame you. There are countless self-help books and experts today that claim to have the definitive answer to what will make you look and feel better. And there's no way to know for sure if their advice is right for you.

I don't claim to have all the answers. But what I can offer you are my own personally tested strategies and tips that have helped *me* look and feel my best over the years. In this book I will share the secrets I've learned from experts I trust—dermatologists, hairdressers, trainers, nutritionists, stylists, doctors, and many more—plus advice from dozens of amazing, beautiful women I admire.

I am still learning ways to better myself, and I hope to continue learning for the rest of my life. I hope your journey brings you to a better place both physically and emotionally. And I hope that this book helps you move through your life with more beauty, grace, and happiness.

Bobbi Brown

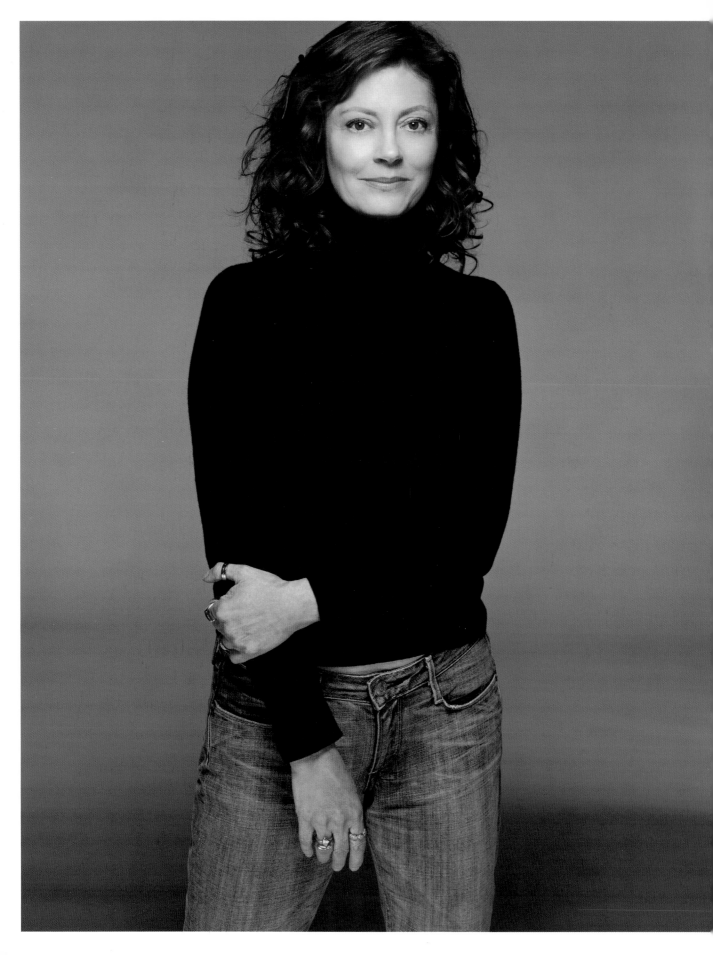

CHAPTER 1

ROLE MODELS

Words of Wisdom from Women Who Have Come of Age Beautifully

I have admired many women over the course of my life—from family members like my mother, grandmother, and Aunt Alice, to silver-screen beauties like Ali MacGraw, Grace Kelly, Sophia Loren, and Audrey Hepburn. As my role models, these women have inspired me and helped me become the person I am today.

When I was about twenty years old, my mom and I saw Goldie Hawn and her children in the lobby of a hotel. Goldie was wearing cool jeans and sneakers, and her kids were dressed to match. She seemed totally comfortable and happy. I made a mental note that I wanted to be that way when I became a mother.

As a freelance makeup artist, I got my fashion inspiration from the magazine editors with whom I worked. They seemed to have it just right. I liked their simple style, hardly there makeup, and big watches (a look I adopted and that is still my trademark today).

When I was thirty years old, I saw a black-and-white picture of Debra Winger in *Rolling Stone* magazine that I thought was amazing. She looked sexy, confident, radiant...but she didn't look like a kid. Her head was tilted back, she had a huge smile on her face, and there were little laugh lines around her eyes and mouth. She looked like the kind of woman I wanted to become. Gazing at Debra's self-assured beauty, I remember saying to myself, "OK, I can do this." The memory of that picture has been with me ever since, and I think of Debra when I look in the mirror now.

All the women featured in this chapter are beautiful—inside and out. They are confident, strong, and charismatic. And most important, they are comfortable in their skin. These women inspire me on many levels, and I hope they inspire you too.

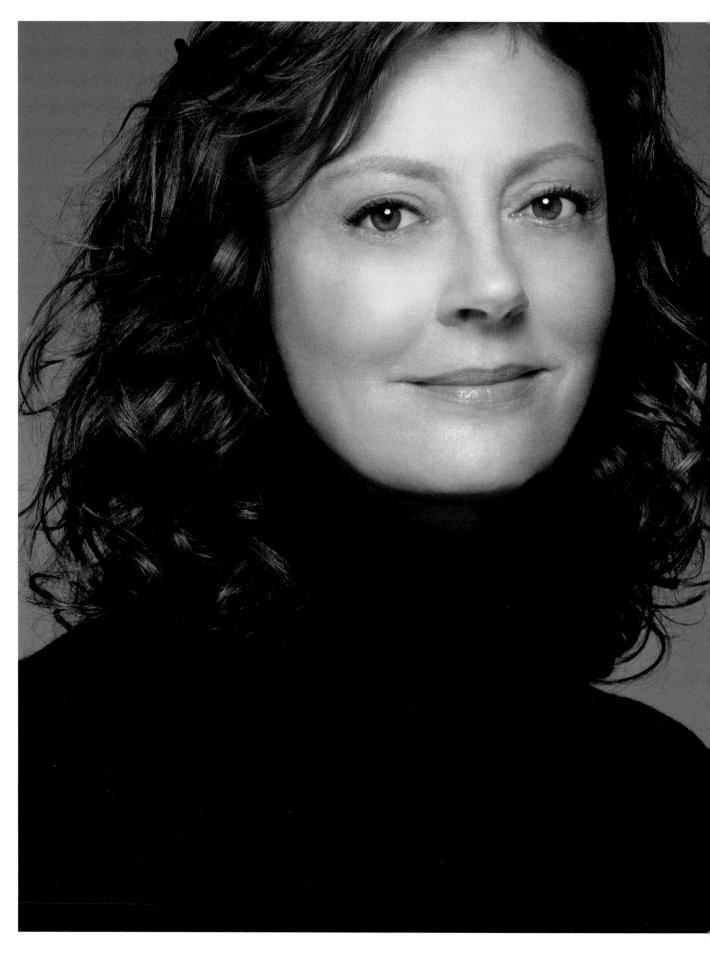

Susan Sarandon on...

...Beauty When I was a kid I sought beauty in perfection. As I got older I began to value the imperfect—for it is there that the unique, the authentic, is manifest. It is there that we see that which makes an individual unique. I am moved by anything that reminds me of the vulnerability of life, and the courage it takes to live.

...Aging "It's not for sissies," to quote Bette Davis.

...Looking Good Not smoking, cardiovascular exercise, greens, and, most important, attitude. When I'm open, joyful, curious, and compassionate, I look my best. Self-love. The realization that age brings wisdom, confidence, and perspective that is palpable and admired by those who are still trying to figure out who they are.

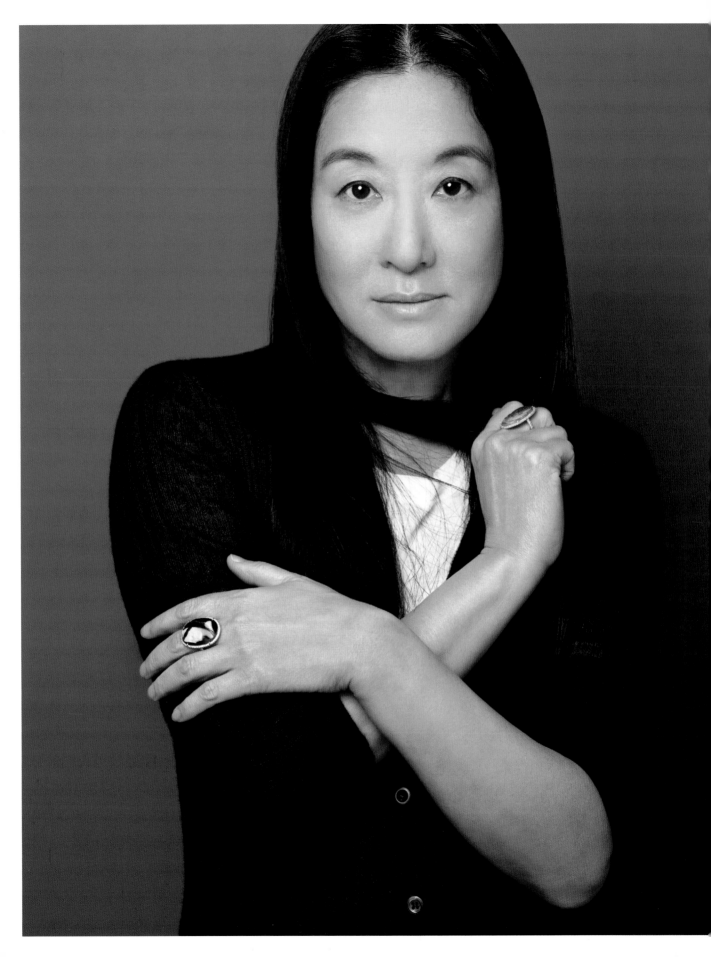

Vera Wang on...

...Beauty It's an artful way of looking at yourself and understanding what will make you feel a little cleaner and neater. Your personality should always come through. Beauty is the thing that makes every face unique...and you should never lose that.

...Aging I have friends in their sixties and seventies whom I consider absolutely beautiful—not because they look young, but because they have maintained their character. They haven't given in to plastic surgery and the idea that you have to fit a certain aesthetic to be beautiful.

...Looking Good My biggest secret is sleep. It's amazing what a few nights of rest do for how my face looks. My other secret weapon is maintaining a healthy (rather than bone-thin) weight. I keep my look very simple and clean. When I do my makeup I focus on evening out my complexion with foundation...it literally takes twenty years off my face. I'm obsessed with skin because it's what we're all packaged in—it's the ultimate accessory.

Lorraine Bracco on...

...Beauty Personality. Someone who is comfortable in her own skin. That's beautiful.

...Aging When I turned fifty, I decided my life motto would be "more fun!" I have had a much younger boyfriend for the past four years....That helps!

...Looking Good I struggled with adult acne for years. It started in my mid-twenties. For years, my dermatologist encouraged me to go on Accutane. After more than five years of consistent breakouts, it was obvious that I had a hormonal imbalance that was often triggered by stress. Despite my doctor's encouragement, I waited almost ten years. I had a lot of mixed feelings about going on medication. When I finally went on it, my skin changed completely. I can't tell you what it did for my confidence and overall well-being. My only regret is that I didn't do it sooner. Keep in mind, medication is not right for everyone, but it's important to know your options. For me, it was the right choice. Also, a good haircut is a great beauty boost!

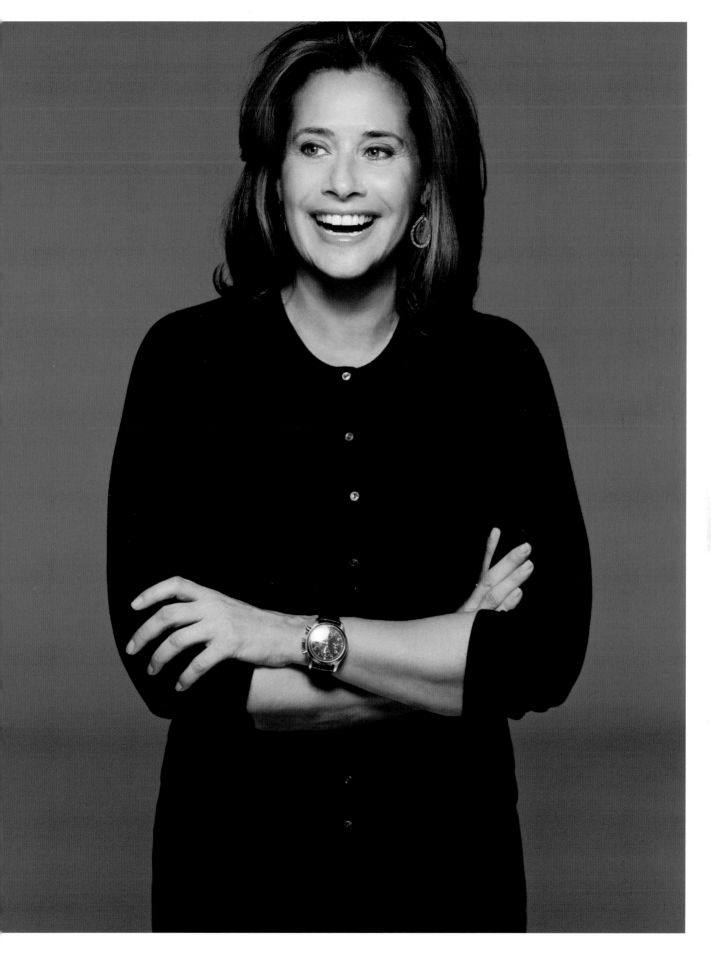

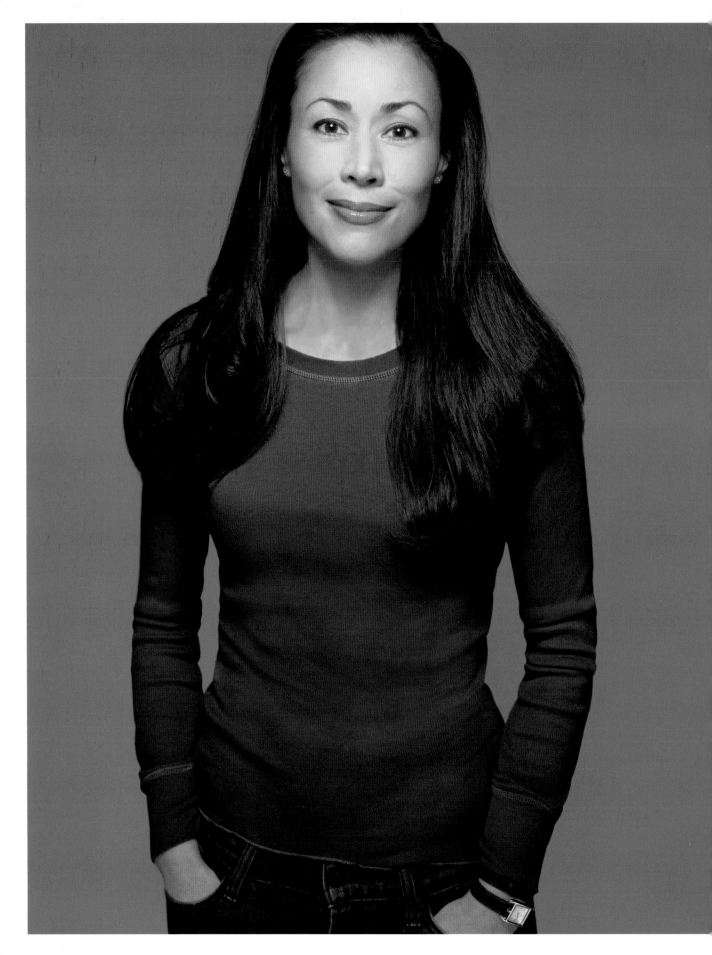

Ann Curry on...

...Beauty Beauty once seemed to me to be an accident of nature. As a young woman I realized it had more to do with ancestry and makeup than anything else, and so I felt oddly disconnected whenever people told me I was beautiful. But now that I can see my life on my face—the suffering in my brow, the joy in the tiny crow's-feet, the confidence in my eyes—I realize we earn the way we end up looking. Time, it seems, gives us all a chance to really be beautiful.

...Aging Isn't it startling, given how much attention we pay to the outside of our bodies, how most of it really comes from the inside? I think we need to make over our minds.

...Looking Good I do eat less bread and sugar, more fresh fruits and vegetables, exercise some, moisturize regularly, and really try to sleep. But above everything else, the thing that helps me make the most of my looks is my daily effort to be a good person. I just feel amazing when I do something useful for other people, and I strive to do so in my personal life and in my news reporting. So even when I am eating the wrong things and not getting enough sleep, I can catch the face of a happy woman in the mirror and feel beautiful.

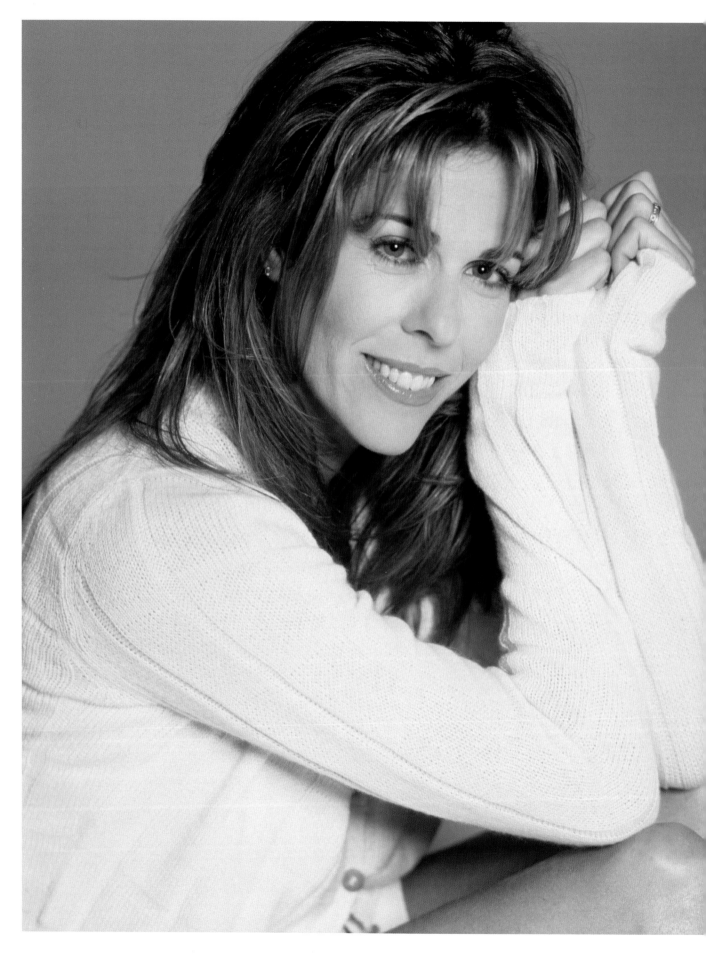

Rita Wilson on...

...Beauty Beauty seems to be more internal now. I respond to someone's spirit, confidence, kindness, and simplicity. It's not that physical beauty, as we have always perceived it, isn't important. To me, that is just one element of what beauty means to me now. I'm attracted to qualities that are more eternal than just the physical aspects.

...Aging I look for inspiration in the many that have gone before me. My mother is a great example of how to age. She is eighty-four, has never had any plastic surgery, and she shares her spirit, her love, her time, and herself at any given moment. Her selflessness teaches me about where to put my energy.

...Looking Good Acceptance. You've got to start there. This has nothing to do with age. When you accept who you are, what you look like, what God's gifts to you are, you can't help but feel liberated.

Marcia Gay Harden on...

...Beauty Beauty is an *attitude*—a perspective that encompasses health, food, skin, makeup, clothing, and *behavior.* Beauty, for me, is extremely removed from glossy magazine photos. Beauty lies in body language, gestures, a smile; beauty is clean, beauty smells good, beauty feels good, beauty is comfortable. Beauty can be exciting and daring.

...Aging I deal with the changes of growing older by completely embracing age. I'm not against minor surgical help if that is what will make someone feel better...a little Botox or wrinkle relief or whatever. But it's silly to try to look twenty when you're forty! I *try* to be beautiful in action and word—it can transform not just the physical (my face or body) but the energy between two people. Part of beauty is being open to change. Part of beauty in your forties is trying to understand the ideas and music of the beauties in their teens!

...Looking Good I always use foundation to even out my skin tone. I have rosacea, and a red nose isn't beautiful. I've recently started using a blush with shine for my cheekbones...it gives me a luminescence that's great. I color my hair as well. While gray is fine for some people, there is no room for it in my life! I also like a few highlights in my hair. Mostly I stick to a healthy diet (lots of raw food) and an exercise program. What you eat changes everything! Also, good posture is the cheapest and most effective beauty plan I can think of.

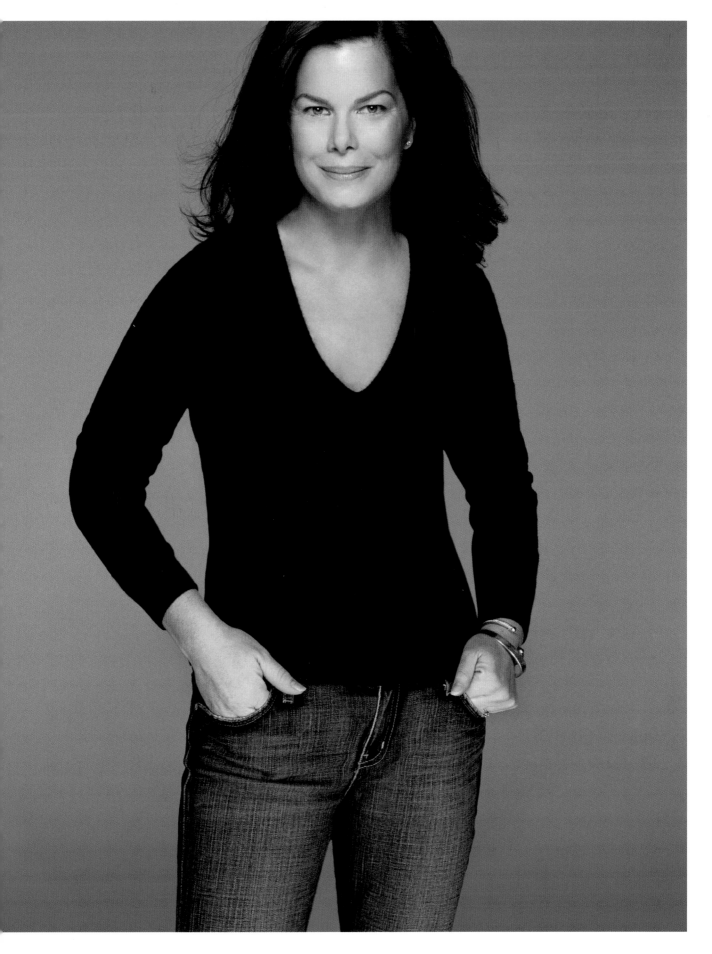

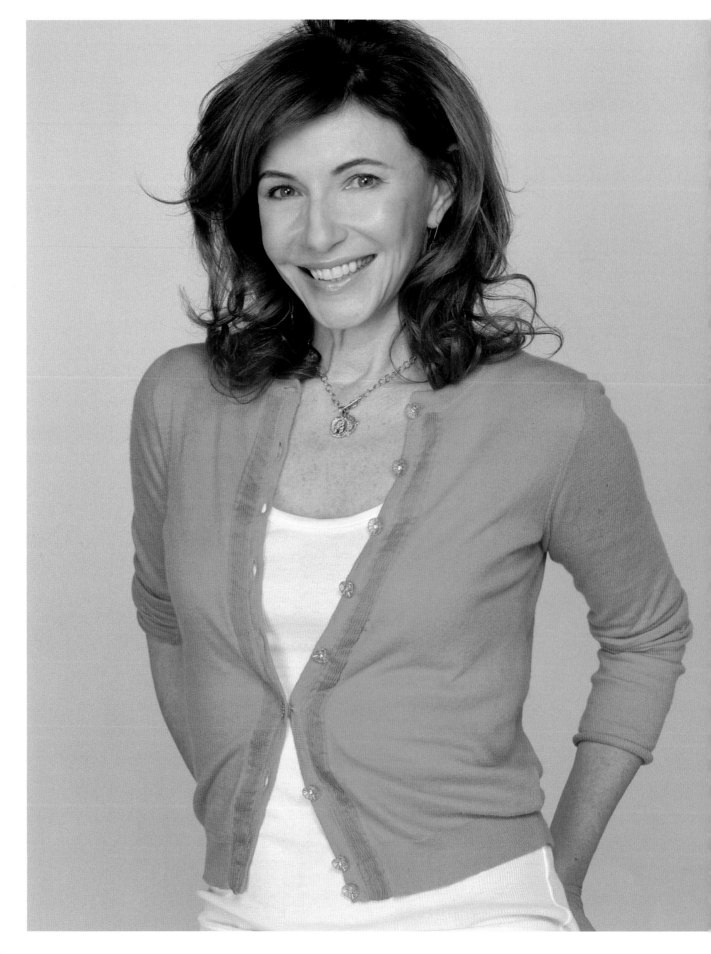

Mary Steenburgen on...

...Beauty A beautiful face is one that belongs to a person who is fulfilling her life's purpose. The details of it are less important than what it speaks to the world of the person inside.

...Aging I have a lot of laugh lines. I treasure every one of them and I hope to have many more before my time is up.

...Looking Good For a very long time I neglected my eyebrows. I've come to realize the importance of beautiful, strong brows. Having the correct shape for your face makes all the difference. I love playing with color, and I realized one day that when I used a dark plum shade of eyeliner, it popped the green in my eyes.

Vanessa Williams on...

...Beauty I think it means being comfortable—comfortable with yourself, your surroundings, and the situations that you encounter. The hardest thing is to stay in the moment and not stress about the future or mourn and regret the past.

...Aging As long as women are empowered, aging is not an obstacle. If you lose all your power because it's based on your beauty, that's when you show your vulnerability. Behind the camera, in front of the camera, and in everyday life, I see so many women in power. I think we're at a great point in terms of embracing our age and having no limitations.

...Looking Good If you have a good skincare regimen, you need less of everything else. I like makeup that makes me look natural and doesn't take longer than ten minutes. I'm good as long as my skin is smooth and hydrated, I've got a smack of lip gloss on, and my brows are done.

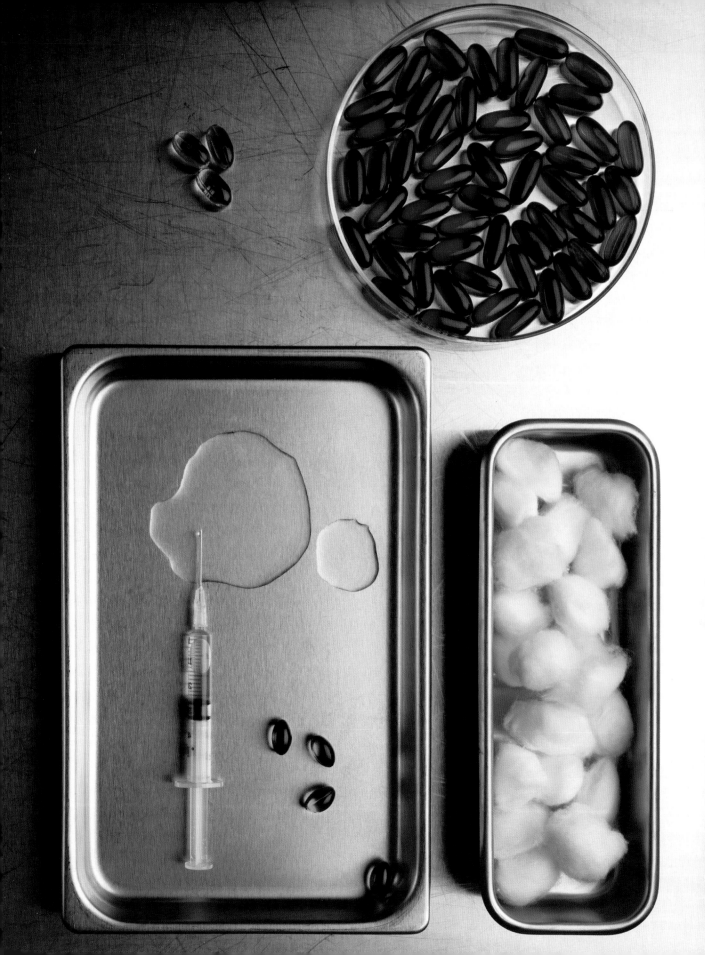

CHAPTER 2

SKIN SAVERS

What a Good Dermatologist Can Do for You

If you're buying this book, you probably know that I'm a makeup artist—not a dermatologist. So why am I writing a chapter about what your dermatologist can do for you? One of my core beliefs is that a beautiful face starts with beautiful skin. And your dermatologist is your partner in attaining and maintaining gorgeous skin—especially as you enter your forties, fifties, and beyond. My goal with this chapter, first and foremost, is to take the mystery out of the nonsurgical options that are available for treating the different skin issues that arise as we get older.

I knew that I'd learn a lot as I started to research this information. But as I began to talk with my dermatologist and other top experts, I realized that the sheer number of treatments out there is totally overwhelming. Adding to the confusion, the experts aren't really in agreement about which treatments work and which don't. Something

touted as "the newest, best thing" by one dermatologist is viewed with skepticism by another. How could I cut through the hype to find the best information?

I started outlining all the options out there—from widely used standard treatments to up-and-coming procedures—and when I was done I couldn't believe my eyes. The outline went on for pages. I realized that if a woman wanted to, she could easily go to the dermatologist every day for a month and try something new each time. A scary—and expensive—proposition. I had visions of women walking around looking like science experiments gone awry, and that didn't sit right with me.

My "aha" moment came one morning while watching a television interview of two famous fifty-something models. One model looked amazing—she had an animated face, bright skin, and tiny

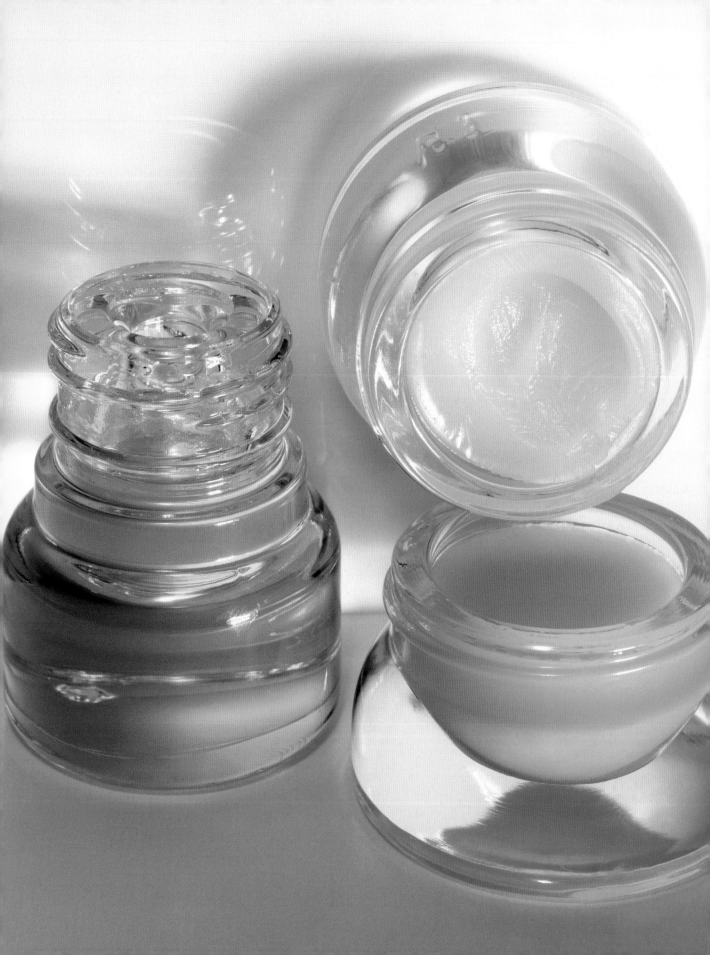

laugh lines around her eyes. She looked happy and beautiful and utterly comfortable in her own skin. The other woman didn't look natural at all—she was totally wrinkle-free, with an immobile expression and no planes in her face at all (most likely the result, I've learned, of too many fillers).

It was at that moment that I figured out exactly what I was going to say in this chapter. I'm not going to tell you to do everything you can to completely erase all the signs of age. *Living Beauty* is about finding the little things that will improve your looks without changing your face and who you are. That's why I've tested and approved every treatment I recommend in this chapter. With the help of my own dermatologist, Dr. Jeanine B. Downie, I will cover only those treatments that I have used myself and believe in 100 percent, with a few noted exceptions. And since not all experiences are the same, I will also share the stories of women who have tried the different treatments and share their results. (Note: These treatments can be expensive. If you're on a budget or paying for your children's college tuition, see Chapter 3 for ways to look fresh without straining your wallet.)

I truly believe that this is just the beginning—and that in the future we're going to see many more options to make ourselves look fresher and better. Just remember that it's not about looking younger; it's about looking as great as you can look for your age.

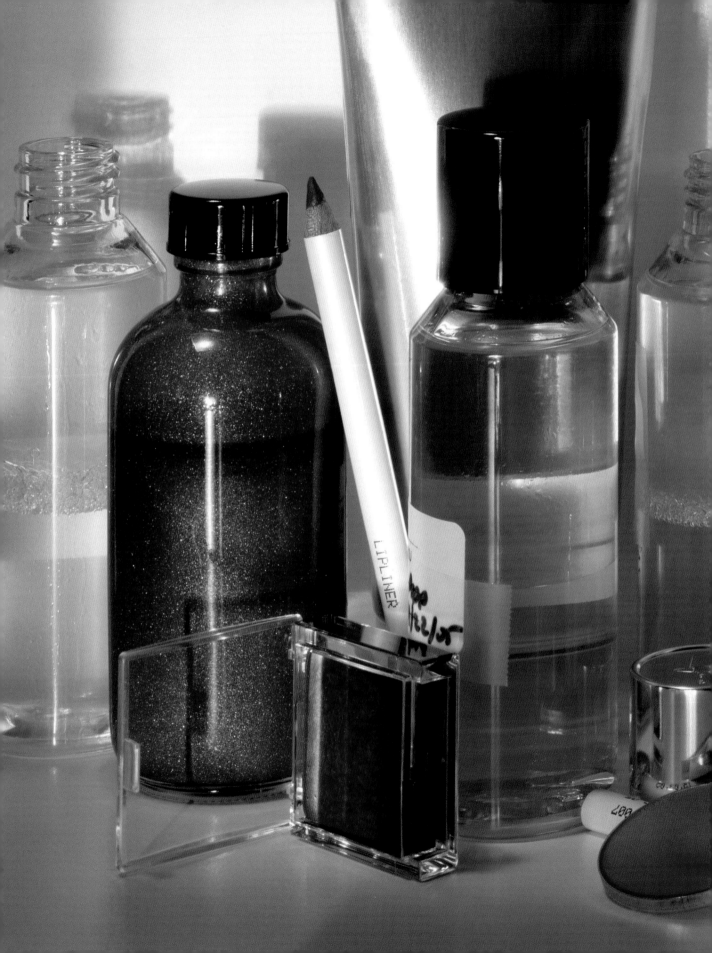

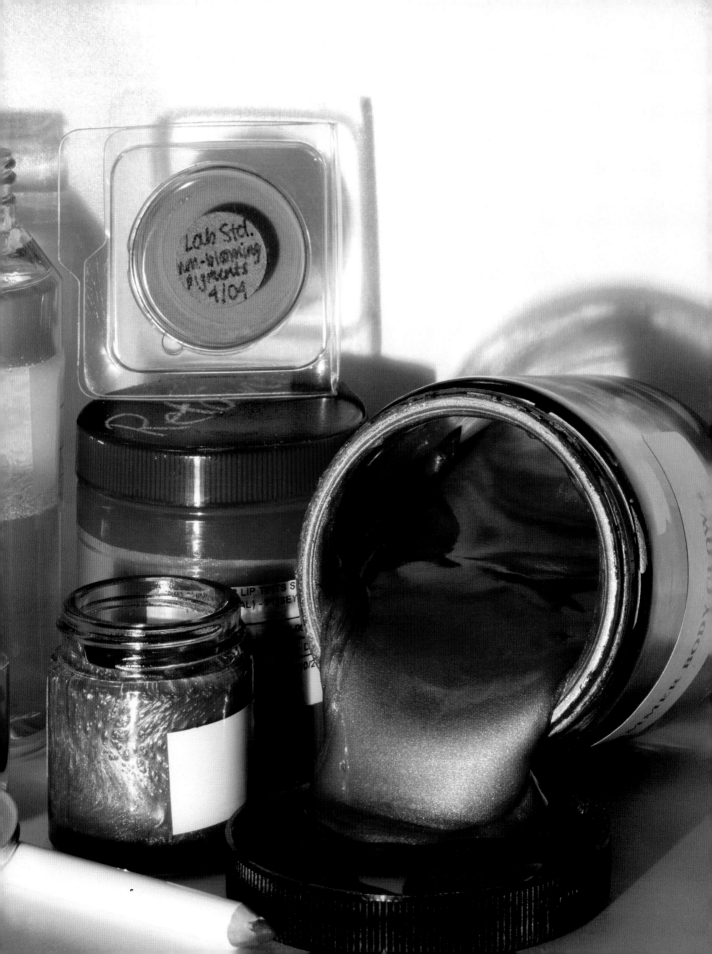

What do you see when you look in the mirror?

As part of the baby-boomer generation, I grew up in an era that equated beauty with suntanned skin. The thinking at the time was "the tanner the better." I spent countless summers in my teens and twenties sunbathing in nothing more than a bikini and a liberal application of baby oil and iodine. If I had known then what I know now about the skin-damaging effects of the sun, I definitely would have covered up.

I've been lucky genetically, but when I look at my skin now I can see the effects of the years I went sunscreen-free. Our skin doesn't lie. When skin isn't well cared for, it shows—particularly when you hit your forties, fifties, and sixties. A few factors impact how skin ages. Genetics plays a big role. Look at the older women in your family for a preview of what you can expect in the years ahead. And the choices you made in the past, especially your sun exposure, will come into play now, too. Too much time in the sun not only breaks down collagen and elastin, but also causes hyperpigmentation (dark spots, also known as age spots). Your lifestyle choices affect skin as well—including how much water you drink (it's important to hydrate skin from the inside out), whether or not you smoke (smoking robs skin of oxygen, affects its elasticity, gives it a dull gray look, and makes dark circles look darker), and how much stress you're under (when I've had a sleepless night, it always shows in my face).

But some skin changes after forty are totally out of our control. Our skin continually sheds dead surface cells and replaces them with new ones, but this process of renewal gradually slows down with age, which is why skin loses its youthful glow. You'll notice some other changes in how your skin looks and feels, too: in your forties, oil production diminishes and skin becomes dryer; collagen breaks down and skin starts to thin; and wrinkles around your eyes and mouth become more noticeable. In your fifties, your skin will bear the effects of menopause—you may notice changes in texture and elasticity; skin may become drier; and you may see irregular pigmentation or the beginnings of rosacea. In your sixties, skin has more wrinkles and it loses a lot of its color and elasticity.

Regardless of what decade you're in, you should wear sunscreen every day. Choose a broad spectrum sunscreen that blocks out both UVA and UVB rays and has an SPF of at least 15. You don't want to avoid the sun, just respect it. (Besides, I still think we look good with a little color on our faces.) Just be sure to stay out of the sun between noon and 4:00 p.m. (the time when sun's rays are most damaging) and wear sunscreen and a hat.

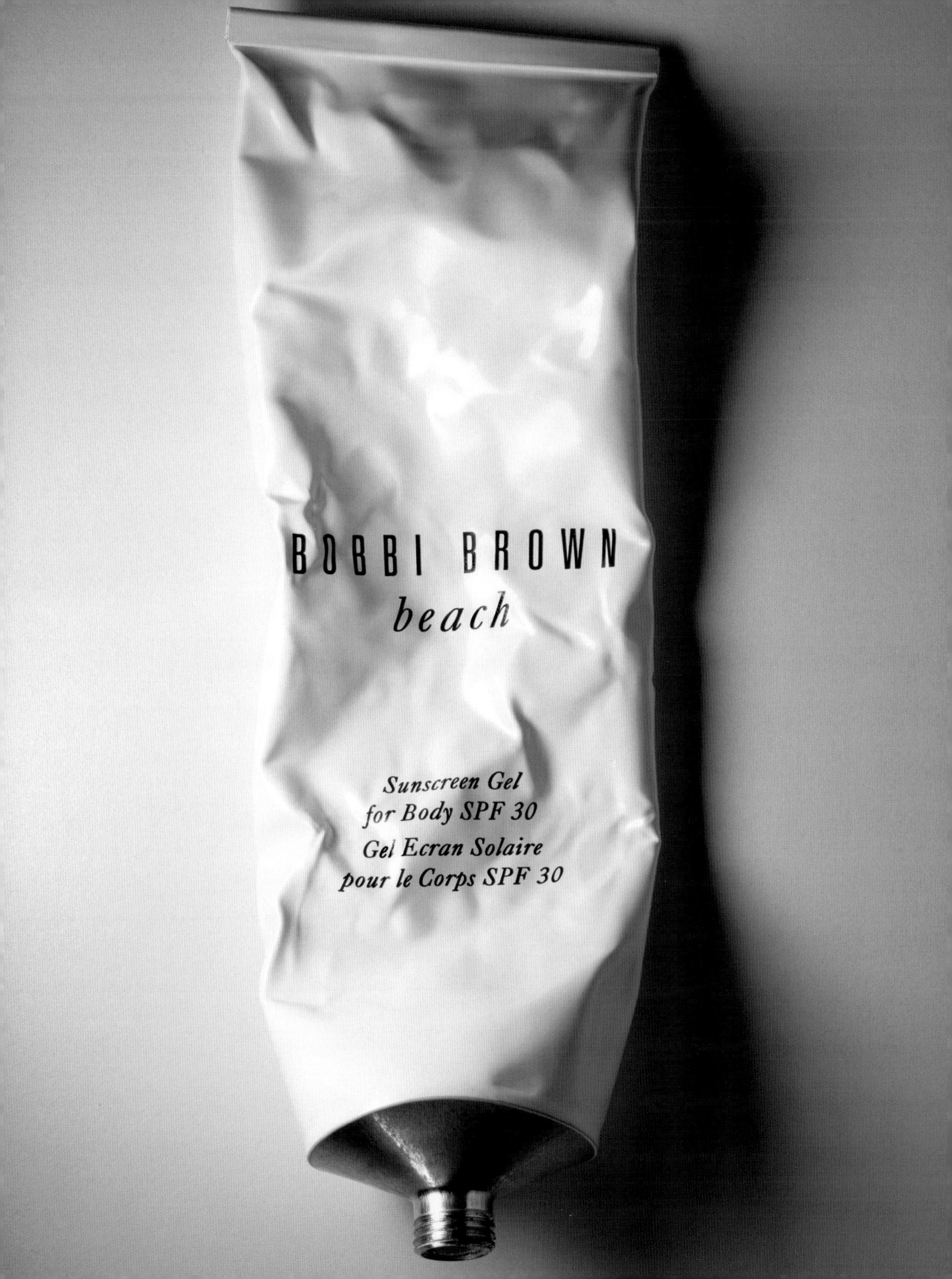
BOBBI BROWN
beach
Sunscreen Gel
for Body SPF 30
Gel Ecran Solaire
pour le Corps SPF 30

How to Soften Expression Lines

When it comes to treating fine lines and wrinkles, I don't believe that there's such a thing as a "miracle" cream. In fact, if it sounds too good to be true, it probably is. And I don't think we should strive to erase every single line we see in our faces—we've earned them and we should wear them with pride (I've actually begun to like the ones that I get around my eyes when I smile). But if you want to diminish the look of some of your lines, there are two topical solutions available today that I truly believe in: growth factors and retinoids.

Growth factors are compounds that stimulate cell regeneration in different parts of the body.

When applied to the skin as a topical cream, growth factors encourage collagen production, which helps soften the look of lines. According to Dr. Downie, growth factors are a good choice if your skin is too sensitive for products containing retinoids or alpha hydroxy acids. Growth factors can be used five times a week for as long as desired. I've tried TNS Recovery Complex and have definitely seen an improvement in the look of my skin.

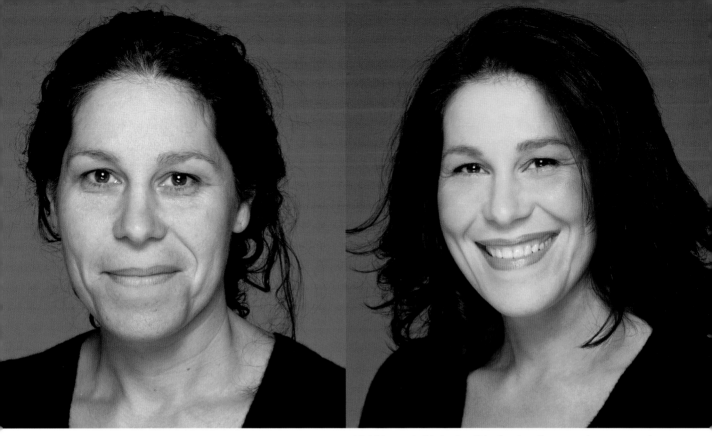

All Athie needed to look polished and pretty was undereye concealer, pinky rose blush, a sheer, deep pink lip color, and a great blow-out.

CASE STUDY: Athie Daniskas

PROFILE: My skin has been all over the map as an adult. I had the best skin during my four pregnancies (I guess it was all the hormonal changes). Since then, I've dealt with breakouts and some discoloration. And while I think lines give you character, I'm not opposed to trying natural, non-surgical ways to help my skin look better. I have extremely sensitive skin, so I'm careful about what I put on my face. I've tried a few different skincare regimens and nothing's worked in the past, so I'm excited to try this treatment.

EXPERIENCE: The first thing Dr. Downie did was to talk to me about the importance of keeping my skin well moisturized and wearing sunscreen every day. Then she instructed me to apply a pea-sized amount of TNS Recovery Complex on my forehead, cheeks, and chin every other night. When I first started the treatment, I felt like everything was coming to the surface and I had redness and some dryness. After a week I noticed some changes in my skin texture. My pores seemed smaller and my skin felt softer.

RESULTS: I've seen a definite improvement in my skin since I started using TNS two months ago. The lines on my forehead and around my eyes are less pronounced. I've even noticed that a pockmark on my temple doesn't seem as deep. TNS is by no means a quick fix. The improvements are gradual. If you're methodical and faithful about applying TNS, eventually you will see the results.

Retinoids, which are vitamin-A derivatives, are another effective way to stimulate collagen production and help renew the skin.

Retinoids can cause some irritation and you may see some dryness and flakiness. Your skin will also become more sensitive to the sun, so it's especially important to protect yourself with a sunscreen of at least SPF 30. And to be truly effective, retinoids must be used over an extended period of time—approximately a month. But I swear I noticed an improvement right away. Topical creams containing retinoids are available by prescription from your dermatologist under brand names like Retin-A Micro and Renova (Renova is the gentler of the two) and can be applied up to twice a week as needed.

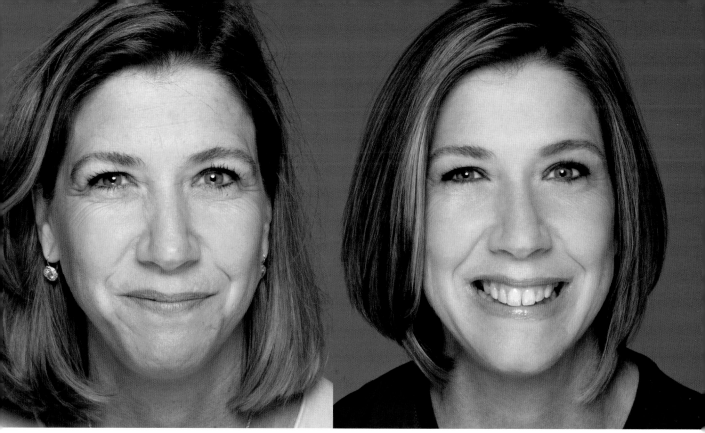

Leslie's beautiful eyes really stand out when they're lined all around with deep navy liner. Foundation smoothes her skin and evens out her complexion.

CASE STUDY: Leslie Larson

PROFILE: I have what I call "colorful" skin—I've got freckles, broken blood vessels, and uneven skin tone. The most noticeable changes in my skin over the years are the appearance of deep forehead lines and extreme dryness. I'm religious about moisturizing and I drink plenty of water, but my skin still feels very tight (it's like my dad's). I'm of the generation that didn't know about all the dangers of sun exposure, so I spent a lot of time in the sun when I was younger. I'm paying for it with sun damage and I'm now diligent about covering up. (I wear sunscreen on a daily basis, and if I'm outdoors for long periods of time, I wear a hat or find shade under an umbrella.)

EXPERIENCE: I applied the retinoid cream every other night and was told to let it sink in for twenty minutes before I followed up with my moisturizer. The first thing I noticed was that I had some dryness and flaking. That subsided about two weeks into the treatment and now my skin is starting to feel smoother, especially on my cheeks.

RESULTS: After a month of using the retinoid cream, I feel like my skin is smoother and the fine lines are not as noticeable. I definitely see an overall improvement, but the deep lines are still there. I think it's important to be realistic about the cream and what it can do for you. You can't reverse the aging process, but you can slow it down a bit. My face is the face of a mature woman and that's OK.

How to Revive Dull Skin

My eye is always drawn to women with glowing skin. In my opinion, there's nothing more beautiful. Young skin glows naturally—you see it in babies, children, even women in their twenties. Unfortunately, this glow does dull with age and it's the result of a slow-down in skin-cell turnover. In addition to exfoliating, I've found that chemical peels are an effective way to encourage the process through which skin renews itself.

Chemical Peel
A peel is basically an acid solution that is applied to the face to remove the dead outermost layer of skin cells.

Not all peels are created equal. At-home peels (the kind you can buy at the drugstore) have the lowest percentage of acid and are so mild that you won't see a tremendous difference in your skin. Spa peels are slightly stronger than their at-home counterparts and shouldn't be done more than once or twice a month. Chemical peels administered by the dermatologist are typically formulated with glycolic acid, salicylic acid, lactic acid, or trichloroacetic acid (TCA). The amount of acid used in the peels can vary from mild (20 percent acid) to deep (99 percent acid) depending on your skin type and what you hope to achieve. Mild peels seldom cause irritation, don't involve downtime, and can be administered once a week. Medium and deep peels cause skin to redden and slough off and it takes about a week for skin to heal fully. Medium peels can be applied every two weeks depending on skin tone. Deep peels should be applied no more than once a month. Skin is especially sensitive after a peel, so it's important to wear sunscreen with an SPF of at least 30.

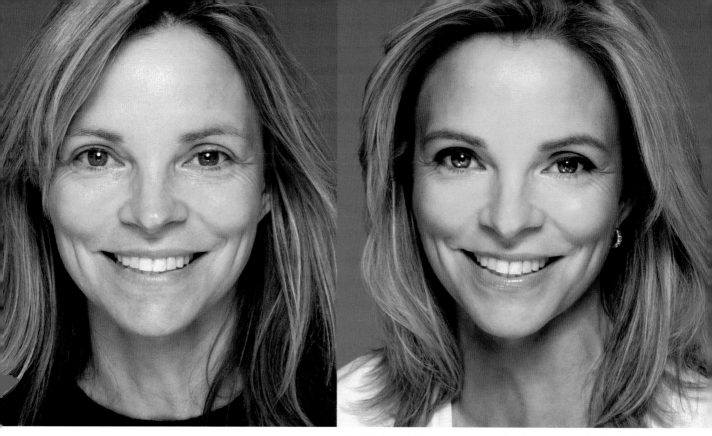

On Julie I used black mascara to define her eyes, blonde shadow to fill in her brows, and pink on her lips and cheeks to make her glow.

CASE STUDY: Julie Jackson

PROFILE: I think what's most startling for a lot of women my age is the difference between how we feel inside (I still feel seventeen!) and what we see when we look in the mirror. The changes happened to me in very subtle ways—I started seeing some age spots, my skin got really dry in the winter, and I was dealing with acne again. I'd like to have as many years of healthy-looking skin as I possibly can, and I'm willing to try treatments that are noninvasive. My biggest concern with the chemical peel is how much downtime I'll have before I can go back to the office. I've also heard that peels can make you break out, so I'm worried that the procedure may have more of a negative effect on my skin.

EXPERIENCE: The actual procedure was quick—it took all of five minutes. The peel solution was swabbed all over my face and I was given a hand-held fan to keep discomfort (like slight tingling) to a minimum during the application.

The solution was rinsed off my face immediately after. Other than a little tightness, the peel doesn't look like it will have any adverse effects (like redness or irritation) on my skin. I'm not going to have any downtime from this treatment, which was my main concern. I'm noticing that some of my pores seem smaller and I'm told that it takes three to four days before you see the full benefit of the peel.

RESULTS: My skin felt a little dry the day after the peel and I had one breakout that went away quickly. Three or four days later, my skin felt and looked great—it was really clear and very smooth. Since getting the peel I've been using less makeup. I don't need as much foundation or color to make my skin look good. Between the zero downtime and the great results, I'd definitely do a peel again.

How to Restore Elasticity

A gradual decrease in skin elasticity is one of the inevitable changes that comes with age. What's to blame for this? Some of the factors are beyond our control, like genetics and lower levels of estrogen in the body (for more information on the effects of estrogen on your skin, see Chapter 6 about menopause). But some of the things that affect skin's elasticity are within our control, like smoking, stress, diet, and sun exposure. Although it may seem easier said than done, try not to stress when things start to go south. Your skin may not be as supple it used to be, but you're certainly smarter, wiser, and more confident (qualities that are far more compelling than anything skin-deep).

Laser Skin Rejuvenation

If you're really bothered by what you see in the mirror, consider non-ablative laser skin rejuvenation.

Here's how it works: high-intensity pulses of light work beneath the skin's surface so there's no visible injury to skin. Skin tissue absorbs this light energy, then "heals" itself by producing new, more elastic collagen. One session takes about fifteen minutes, and you can expect to see improvement after three to five treatments, spaced every three to four weeks. This procedure won't give you the skin of your twenty-something years, but it can help tighten and tone things. Skin is more sensitive to sun after the treatment, so be sure to wear sunscreen. In addition to improving overall skin tone, laser skin rejuvenation can also help reduce ruddiness.

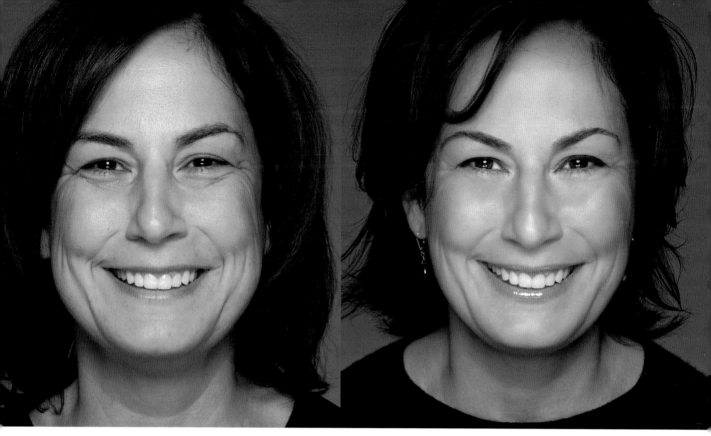

Giving Amy a layered haircut instantly updated her look. A bit of black eyeliner made her eyes sparkle and completed her makeover.

CASE STUDY: Amy Rosen

PROFILE: Turning fifty got me thinking about new milestones in my life. I've been really lucky in that I've always had good skin, and I've kept my skincare regimen pretty simple with a mild cleanser and moisturizer. I did spend far too much time in the sun as a young adult, although up until recently I felt like I wasn't paying the price for it. But now I'm seeing some brown spots. In the last five years my skin has really dried out and everything is a little looser than it used to be. I have a bit of blotchiness and I've just started using foundation to help cover it up. Dermatologists offer so many treatments today that if you're not paying attention, it's easy to go overboard with a little bit of this and a little bit of that. At fifty I don't want to be trying to look thirty.

EXPERIENCE: I went in for a series of four laser treatments, each lasting less than ten minutes. Dr. Downie applied some gel to my face and rolled a wand over the areas where I had broken blood vessels. I experienced a light prickling sensation. What I liked about the treatment was that it was so subtle and my skin didn't feel like it was being overly manipulated. I felt like this wasn't something that was going to cause bruising or noticeable damage to my skin.

RESULTS: I left each of the sessions feeling like I looked better. I couldn't quite define what was better because the differences were so subtle, but they were definitely there. My complexion looks better than it has in a long time. My nose and cheeks aren't as red as they used to be, so I don't need to use foundation to even out my complexion. The sunspots that I had are now gone. And that's what I love the most about getting the laser treatments. The spots were the first thing I saw when I looked in the rearview mirror, and not seeing them now makes my day. At the end of four treatments I see how I could get hooked on this.

How to Erase Brown Spots

Brown spots—also referred to as sunspots, age spots, and even worse, liver spots—are the result of a combination of factors: sunbathing for hours on end with little or no sun protection, natural fluctuations in hormone levels (from birth control pills, pregnancy, and menopause), and genetics. I started noticing brown spots in my late thirties and have tried removing them with both skin-bleaching products and laser resurfacing. Skin-bleaching products contain hydroquinone, an antioxidant that helps suppress the enzymes in the skin responsible for producing melanin. Over-the-counter products, which contain 2 percent hydroquinone, may help lighten spots slightly. Products with a 4 percent hydroquinone preparation, which are available by prescription only, are said to be far more effective. I tried a cream that combined 4 percent hydroquinone, a topical steroid, and tretinoin, a vitamin-A derivative, for a few months and didn't see a noticeable difference in the color of the spots.

Laser Resurfacing In my opinion, there's nothing more effective in removing brown spots than ablative laser resurfacing.

Ablative lasers essentially target the melanin (a pigment that gives color to the skin) and blast it to smithereens. A topical numbing cream is applied before the procedure to keep discomfort to a minimum, then the laser heats and removes the top layer of tissue. Small scabs form shortly after the treatment and when they fall off, they reveal spot-free skin (though some stubborn spots may need repeat procedures to fade away completely). Lasered skin is more sensitive to the sun, so it's important to cover up with a broad-spectrum sunscreen formulated with at least SPF 30.

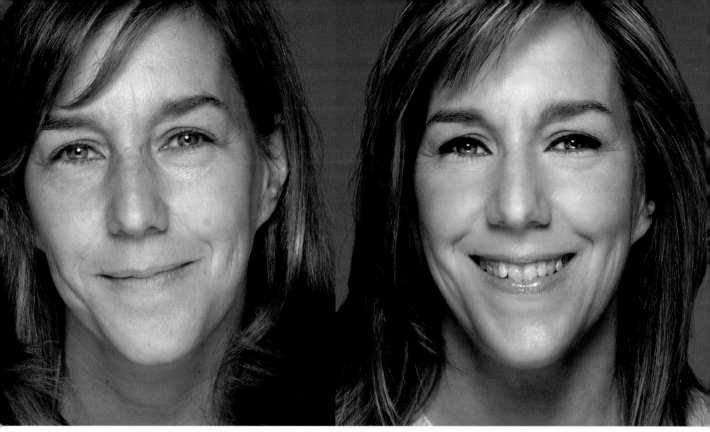

I used pink blush and petal lip gloss to lift and brighten Naomi's face, while still keeping her look natural.

CASE STUDY: Naomi Drewitz

PROFILE: First I saw my grandmother develop brown spots on her face, then I saw my mom get them—and I still thought it wouldn't happen to me. I was in my early thirties when I got my first brown spots. They started on my hands and arms, then appeared on my face. I hated the spots because I thought they made me look older than I felt. I tried everything to cover them up—from makeup to a high-intensity vitamin E cream from the health food store. Over the course of the last five years I've started staying out of the sun to prevent the appearance of more brown spots. I'm looking forward to trying laser resurfacing and I'm not worried about the pain or discomfort during the procedure. What I am worried about is what I'll look like immediately after the procedure, how I'll heal, and if there will be any scarring.

EXPERIENCE: The actual procedure was OK and took about twenty minutes to complete. Dr. Downie used what looked like a little pen to burn spots off my face and chest. When I walked out of the office it didn't look like anything had been done. Within two hours the treated spots turned pink and by that night they were brown. The following morning scabs started to form. After a few more days, the scabs turned dark brown and became very itchy. Dr. Downie told me to keep the spots moisturized with Vaseline and to wear sunscreen with an SPF 30 all the time. The hardest part was not picking or rubbing the spots.

RESULTS: The scabs eventually shrank and basically dissipated. I have to say I was pleasantly surprised by how well the healing went. Not all the brown spots disappeared entirely, but they all faded. The most prominent spot on my cheek—the one that bothered me the most—is much lighter, and all the spots on my chest are now clear. The overall effect is great. When you have brown spots you just get used to seeing them and you don't realize how different you can look without them. It's a cleaner, more refreshed look.

Spa Facials
An Interview with Marcia Kilgore

I've always loved going to the spa because it's one of the few places where I slow down long enough to keep my thoughts from racing a mile a minute. During a recent trip to Telluride, I treated myself to an oxygen facial. My face was misted with pure oxygen gas, which is said to help improve circulation and stimulate cell repair. I'm not sure if the facial impacted my skin on a cellular level, but I do know that my skin felt great and had more of a glow immediately after.

Spa-goers and spa experts all have different opinions on the benefits of facials. For some, facials are a way to feel pampered and relaxed. Others view facials in more pragmatic terms—as a necessary part of a good skincare regimen. I chatted with Marcia Kilgore, founder and creative director of the popular Bliss Spa, to get her expert take on facials.

Bobbi—What are the benefits of facials? Marcia—In the world as it is today, we're so rushed that it's a real luxury to do something that's just for you—where the phones aren't ringing, the kids aren't yelling, and your boyfriend or husband isn't asking you for something. Facials make you feel better because they're incredibly relaxing. And then there are the countless benefits that facials have on the skin. Facials that include microdermabrasion are regenerating because they take off the dead surface layer of the skin to reveal fresh, smooth skin. This also stimulates lymphatic drainage, which helps the skin rid itself of toxins.

As we get older, our capillary walls become less permeable (because of physiological aging, sun damage, and smoking), which means there's less blood flow into skin tissue cells. An oxygenating facial has a massaging effect on the skin, which unblocks capillaries and makes them better able to deliver nutrients to skin cells. One of the main focuses of facials is cleaning the pores out. This is important because pores are the largest pathway of penetration into the skin for active ingredients (from skincare products) and oxygen in the environment. When pores are clear you're also less likely to break out because you don't have an anaerobic environment where bacteria can flourish.

Bobbi—How often should women get facials? Marcia—Ideally, every four to six months. Even once a year will benefit your skin. If you can't get to a spa, it's not difficult to give yourself an at-home minifacial. Put a warm towel compress over your face and gently press your pores through the towel (whatever you do, never pick at your face with your nails). To give your skin a glow, exfoliate with a mix of fresh orange juice and baking soda. Be sure to rinse the mixture off immediately to prevent irritation.

Bobbi—What can a woman do to maintain her skin in between facials? Marcia—A basic skincare regimen is important. Choose a gentle cleanser that breaks down excess sebum, hydrate skin to prevent trans-epidermal water loss, and wear sunscreen every day (sun damage accounts for 90 percent of the aging that you see in your face). Exfoliate in the shower three times a week to get rid of dead surface skin cells. Be gentle with your skin—more is not necessarily better.

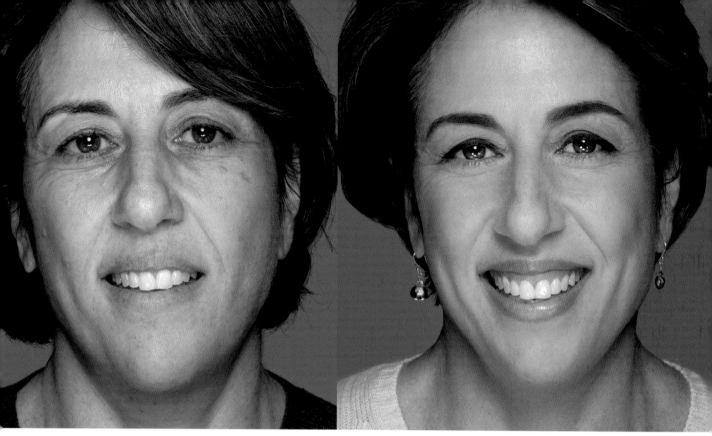

To smooth Amy's skin, I used a warm shade of foundation. Nectar blush on the apples of her cheeks gave her a pretty glow.

CASE STUDY: Amy Lazarus

PROFILE: I have sensitive skin that tends to flare up about once a year. I spent a lot of time in the sun when I was younger, so I have a lot of stubborn spots that even laser treatments haven't been able to remove. Aging didn't bother me when I turned forty, but it really smacked me in the face after forty-five. I'm not thrilled about getting older, but I don't obsess about it either. I've had a few facials, and in general, I haven't seen a dramatic improvement in my skin. In my experience, facials are a good way to feel relaxed and rejuvenated.

EXPERIENCE: I went to Bliss Spa for their Steep Clean facial that included microdermabrasion, massage, pore extraction, and a calming mask. The microdermabrasion wasn't all that pleasant—it felt like sandpaper was being rubbed on my skin and I was worried that I'd emerge red and blotchy. After cleaning out my pores, the aesthetician applied a face mask, which was re-

ally soothing (and I'm sure the relaxing music and lying under a heated blanket helped too!).

RESULTS: After having my face worked on for so long I was concerned that my skin would look irritated. I was pleasantly surprised to see no redness whatsoever after the facial. My skin felt and looked rejuvenated for a few days after, and even my husband said that I looked refreshed. The aesthetician gave me some good pointers on things I could do to improve my skincare regimen (she suggested a different cleanser because the one I was using wasn't removing my makeup thoroughly, a more emollient moisturizer, and a bleaching cream for my sunspots). I think tweaking my skincare routine has also helped.

Botox can help soften expression lines on the face, is the one treatment I'm most conflicted about.

BOTOX: LESS IS MORE

◆

If you decide on Botox, start with less—you can always repeat the process. And remember, a bad job takes a long time to reverse. I think Botox in small doses between the brows and on parts of the forehead can look natural (the idea is to still have movement in your face). Collagen-injected lips, line fillers like Restylane and Captique, and Botox anywhere else—these things never look good.

While I'm against putting unnecessary chemicals into my body, a small amount of Botox can work wonders. I know more women than not who get Botox. Botox is controversial because it is a derivative of a bacteria containing the same toxin that causes food poisoning. However, experts say that this purified protein doesn't stay in the body and that you can't get botulism from Botox injections.

Botox works by relaxing facial muscles so that they can't contract. The approximately ten-minute treatment consists of a series of little injections that feel like tiny pinches or slight stings. Both Dr. Downie and I agree that when it comes to Botox, less is more. The frozen look is passé, and today the aim is to achieve a more natural look that still allows the face to move. You'll see results in seven to ten days, and the effect can last three to four months. If you decide to go for this procedure, make sure you visit a board-certified doctor. Don't go to a spa or Botox party—this is definitely an instance where the adage "You get what you pay for" is true. When Botox is applied incorrectly by unskilled hands, it can freeze one or both of your eyebrows, resulting in a surprised look, or give you a droopy eyelid (the result of injecting the wrong muscle

Nonsurgical "Face-lifts" — Too Good to Be True?

Going under the knife may someday become a thing of the past thanks to a crop of new surgery-free treatments that promise to tone and tighten the face. While there's not enough research to prove their effectiveness, I think these procedures are ones to watch. If they can make you look better and well rested—and not look like "Oh, she's had something done"—I'm all for them.

Acupuncture Facial

Hair-thin needles are inserted into specific points on the face and scalp. The needles cause the underlying muscles to contract or relax. You'll need quite a few sessions to see some results (a course of 8–12 weekly sessions is often recommended).

Thermage

This procedure uses radio frequency to tighten and tone skin. A small metal circle or plate emits radio-frequency waves, which are absorbed by the skin. Heat created by the frequency causes the collagen to tighten. Thermage works well on people who have very little loss of elasticity to begin with. People with a lot of sagging are often disappointed by the slight improvements. You'll most likely need once-monthly treatments over several months (two to six months) to see any changes.

Titan

This is the newest entry in the laser light therapy category of treatments. Infrared light heats the dermis below the skin's surface. This causes collagen in the skin to contract and tighten and also encourages the growth of new, more elastic collagen. Titan is not a quick fix—it may take once-monthly treatments over a period of three to six months before you see an improvement.

Skincare Glossary: Ingredients You Should Know

Whenever I browse the skincare section at the drugstore or department store, I feel like I'm in high school chemistry class. Skincare products today are loaded with all sorts of ingredients that claim to improve the skin both inside and out.

Some claims are based on solid evidence, while other claims stretch the truth. I believe every woman should be her own skincare expert—and this includes knowing how different ingredients work. Here's a look at some of the ones we hear and read about most often.

Alpha hydroxy acids (AHAs) are naturally occurring acids that help loosen up dead surface cells and speed up the skin's natural exfoliation process. AHAs are found in dairy products (lactic acid), sugar (glycolic acid), and citrus fruits (citric acid). Applied topically, AHAs help diminish the look of fine lines and unclog pores.

Antioxidants protect skin from damaging free radicals (also known as oxidants). Free radicals are unstable molecules caused by pollution, smoke, ultraviolet light, and other environmental factors. These unstable molecules attack the skin, causing visible signs of aging like fine lines and wrinkles. Some antioxidants include vitamin C (helps reduce appearance of hyperpigmentation), vitamin E (found in many moisturizers because it makes skin softer and smoother), and green tea (found in many antiaging products).

Ceramides prevent water loss and help encourage skin-cell renewal. They help as a first line of defense for dry, chapped, cracked skin and are found in many over-the-counter moisturizers.

Collagen, a protein found naturally in the skin, is thought to be an effective water-binding ingredient when it's applied topically. Experts differ in opinion on whether creams formulated with collagen can also help boost the skin's ability to produce collagen.

Copper is thought by some experts to help encourage the production of collagen and elastin, two supporting structures in the skin. It's also said to speed up wound healing, but the jury is still out on its effectiveness.

Glycolics are part of the alpha hydroxy acid family. They help speed up the process through which skin sloughs off its outermost layer of dead cells to reveal a layer of new, smooth skin cells.

Growth factors control cell growth in different parts of the body and are used in antiaging creams to help build collagen and soften fine lines and wrinkles. TNS Recovery Complex, a type of growth factor, is a good choice if you have sensitive skin and can't use retinoids or alpha hydroxy acids.

Hyaluronic acid, a sugar molecule, is an ingredient in many moisturizers because it helps skin retain moisture and gives the skin a smoother look.

Hydroquinone is an antioxidant that helps suppress the enzymes in the skin that are responsible for producing pigment. Skincare products containing hydroquinone are recommended by some dermatologists to lighten age spots and dark spots.

Retinoids are vitamin-A derivatives that stimulate collagen production and help renew the skin. Retinoids are also prescribed for the treatment of acne because they help unclog clogged pores. Topical creams like Retin-A Micro and Renova (both available by prescription only) contain retinoids.

Soy isoflavones are thought by some experts to block the pathway of melanin, which might make it helpful in treating dark spots. A type of plant hormone, soy isoflavones also have an effect on skin similar to estrogen and may help prevent collagen loss in postmenopausal women.

Rx SMARTS: MEDICINES COMMONLY PRESCRIBED BY DERMATOLOGISTS

SYMPTOM	R_x
Flaking scalp (dandruff)	OLUX Foam
Dry, excessively chapped lips	Cutivate Ointment
Dry, cracked skin on body (especially feet)	Salex Cream
Acne	Differin Cream
Dark spots and stubborn blemishes	Tri-Luma Cream
Fine lines and wrinkles	Renova

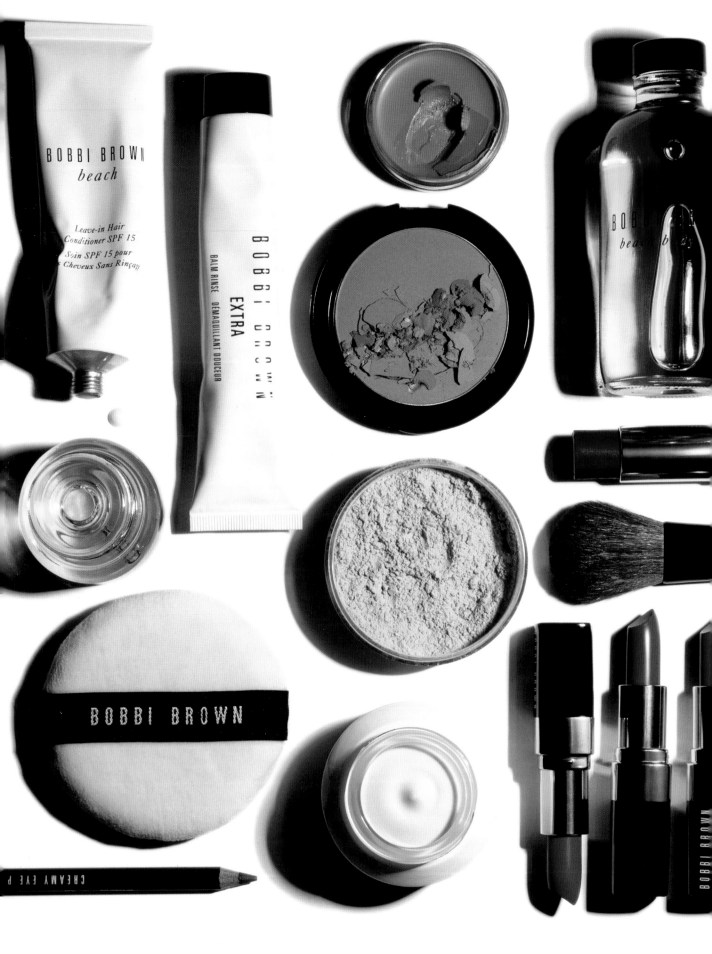

CHAPTER 3

THE MAKEUP FACE-LIFT

Surgery-Free Ways to Wipe Away the Years

I was thirty years old when I discovered that make-up could have the same (or better) effect on a woman's face as a face-lift. Gail, a close friend of mine, was about to turn forty. She was fretting about her upcoming birthday and depressed by what she considered the beginning of her "physical demise." Even though we were ten years apart in age, I had never thought of Gail as an older woman—I only thought of her as totally beautiful. Gail told me that she was considering plastic surgery and was making appointments for consultations with all the best surgeons. I felt strongly that Gail just needed the right makeup to freshen up her look. So I insisted that she visit me at the Frederic Fekkai Salon, where I was the resident makeup artist.

Gail agreed to stop by. Before picking up any of my brushes or makeup, I sat Gail down in a chair and asked her to tell me what was bothering her about her face. She complained about her falling eyelids. (Yes, she did have bedroom eyes, but I thought they were beautiful in an Elvis or a Charlotte Rampling kind of way.) Next, Gail pointed out her sagging skin (honestly, I didn't see what she was talking about) and sallow complexion (OK, her tan was fading). When Gail was done with her rant, I stepped back to take in her face, then I began my work.

First I focused on Gail's skin. To lessen the look of her fine lines and give her skin a smoother, plumped-up look, I gently applied a quick-absorbing eye cream, a hydrating face moisturizer, and a touch of rich face balm. I lightened the darkness under her eyes with just the right combination of concealers, making sure to apply the concealer as close to her lashes as possible and into the inner corner of her eye socket. Next, I smoothed on tinted moisturizer, followed by stick foundation only on the parts of her face that were uneven (around her nose and mouth and the sides of her face). I counteracted her sallow coloring with a medium bronzer on her cheeks, forehead, nose, and neck.

Now that her skin looked flawless, I moved on to the fun part of the process—using makeup to lift her features. I softly filled in her eyebrows with soft blond shadow to lift them, and used a combination of bone eye shadow (dusted all over the lid), taupe eye shadow (smudged on the lower lid), and soft contour shadow (applied to the sides of the eyelid crease) to lift the eyes and give them more definition. Next, I lined her bright blue eyes with a navy shadow to bring them out. I finished off her eyes by curling her lashes and brushing on two coats of rich, very black mascara. I applied a pop of bright pink blush on the apples of Gail's cheeks, then patted a bit of balm on top to give her a glow—and take her attention away from the lines that bugged her. The last step was a pinky nude lipstick, lip pencil, and a soft pink gloss on Gail's lips. I handed Gail a mirror so that she could look at what I had done. After a few seconds, she said exactly what I had hoped she would: "Oh my god. It's like an instant face-lift." (I haven't seen Gail in fifteen years and I'm sure she's still a beauty.)

When I turned forty, I discovered firsthand the tremendous difference makeup makes. Since everything falls and fades, the trick is to lift and add life back to your face with the right textures and colors and use the correct techniques. Because I've figured out how to care for my skin and I've picked up some great makeup tips along the way, I've never (not even for a second) thought about resorting to a face-lift.

In the previous chapter, with the help of dermatologist, Dr. Jeanine Downie, I shared with you what skin treatments actually work for me and make me look better (but still like me). Now, in this chapter, I'll show you what I think are the most effective skincare and makeup solutions for the beauty woes that we encounter as we get older.

BOBBI'S FIVE INSTANT LOOK-LIFTERS

PLUMP

Layer skincare formulas (a wet, hydrating cream under a rich, dense balm) to give skin a plumped-up, cushiony look. Use the warmth of your fingers to help blend the creams.

BRIGHTEN

Lighten the under-eye area and draw your attention up with a pink- or peach-toned corrective concealer paired with a yellow-toned concealer. Be sure to apply concealer close to the lashes and to the inner corner of the eye as well.

POP

Dust blush high on the apples of your cheeks.

DEFINE

When lining eyes, extend the liner ever so slightly at the outer corner of the eye. Make sure the liner is thick enough and visible when your eyes are open.

FINISH

After applying lipstick and pencil, layer a light shade of light-reflecting, high-shine lip gloss on top.

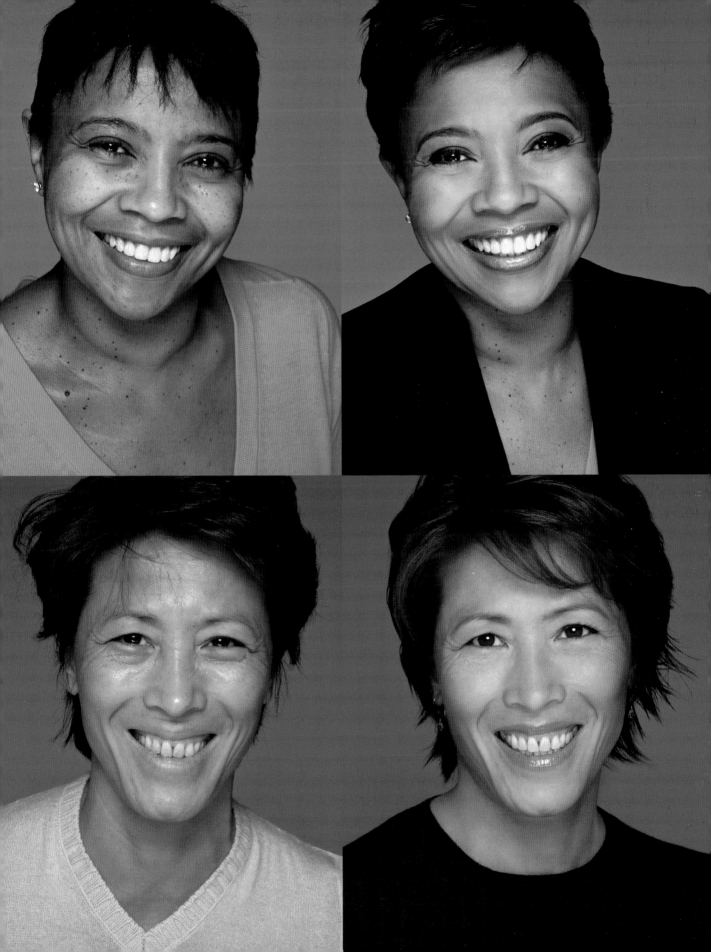

From Barefaced to Beautiful

How to Care for Skin

A good beauty routine should always start with skincare. When skin isn't properly cleansed and hydrated, it shows. A lot of factors play into how skin looks and feels. In addition to genetics, you must pay attention to your diet, the weather, and how much stress you're under. This means that your skin's needs may change on a daily basis— one day your skin may feel very dry, and the next day it might feel normal. So rather than reaching blindly for the same skincare products, learn how to gauge what your skin needs and adjust your routine accordingly.

The Basics

These basic products should be a part of your everyday regimen:

Cleanser If your complexion feels dry, use a cream- or oil-based cleanser that moisturizes as it cleanses. Look for ingredients like wheat germ oil, which cleans without stripping, and glycerin, which attracts moisture to the skin's surface. Water-based gel cleansers with oil-fighting ingredients like seaweed extract are perfect for times when skin feels oily. Ideally, you should have two cleansers: one for days when skin is a bit oilier than normal or needs extra cleaning, and another for days when skin feels a bit drier. Never use body soap on your face, as it will strip skin and leave it feeling tight and dry.

Sunscreen I firmly believe in wearing SPF year-round, not just in the summer. A lotion with SPF protection of 15 to 25 is essential whenever you're outdoors, running errands, or going to work. If you plan on spending an extended amount of time in the sun, cover up with SPF 30 to 50. Apply sunscreen before moisturizer and makeup. Here's a good timesaver: moisturizer with sunscreen is just as effective for daily use.

Moisturizer This is the most important step to look fresher, with or without makeup. When skin isn't well moisturized, it looks dull, tired, and older than it really is. Choose a lightweight moisturizing lotion for everyday use, and opt for a richer, hydrating cream with ingredients like petrolatum, glycerin, or shea butter when your skin feels drier. Even oily skin benefits from moisturizer, so choose an oil-free formula that hydrates while it helps control overactive oil production. Pamper skin overnight with a rich, restorative cream. Don't be afraid of face oil—it's an instant lifter. And experiment with layering formulas, for example, a hydrating cream with a richer balm or face oil.

Eye cream The skin around the eyes is more delicate than the rest of your face and has special needs. In the morning (before you apply concealer), use a lightweight eye cream (it should feel wet) that hydrates and absorbs into skin, leaving it smooth. At night, choose a richer balm containing shea butter or beeswax that will stay on longer and keep hydrating while you sleep.

The Extras

Think of these products as add-ons for when your skin acts up and needs a little something extra:

Toners If skin feels too oily or you're wearing a lot of makeup, a toner can clean away anything your cleanser has left behind. The newest formulas are alcohol-free and don't strip skin of its necessary oils.

Masks Clay masks draw out dirt and impurities from pores. Hydrating masks with glycerin or essential oils add moisture back to skin and leave it feeling soft. Glycolic acid masks and grainy masks exfoliate skin and help unclog pores. For an at-home spa treat, smooth on a mask once a week. You can use different types of masks to pamper your skin and to treat different symptoms.

Serums These concentrated liquids are typically packed with vitamin C and other skin-nourishing nutrients that work to improve skin's appearance and help prevent visible signs of aging. Apply after cleansing, before moisturizer.

Balms I'm never without a balm. These super-rich moisturizers target dry patches of skin on face, hands, feet, and body. Look for thick, dense formulas with ingredients like avocado extract and shea butter. For subtle glow, I warm some in my hands and pat it on my cheeks after applying all my makeup.

Exfoliators These are designed to help slough off dead skin cells. Exfoliate one to two times a week with a scrub that's gentle and designed specifically for the face.

Face oils These are old-fashioned beauty products that work great on dry skin and don't clog pores. I don't care what most dermatologists say—as a beauty expert, I highly recommend using face oils containing sesame, sweet almond, olive, and jojoba oils.

How to Wield a Brush Like a Pro

Any makeup artist will tell you that the right brushes are just as important as the makeup itself. Depending on where you go, you can spend anywhere from under £5 to over £30 on one brush. In general, the brushes sold by makeup artist lines are the best quality and worth the investment. If you're willing to do some legwork, you can also find good brushes for less money in drugstores, beauty supply stores, even art supply stores.

There are a few things you should look for in a brush, regardless of where you shop. The bristles should feel soft against your skin, not scratchy or rough. Try the brush by running it across the part of the face that it's designed for to see how it feels; this is more important than whether it's made of natural or synthetic material. Run your hand through the bristles to make sure they don't come out easily. Brushes sometimes come in different handle lengths, so hold the brush in your hand and make sure it feels comfortable.

These basic brushes are a good place to start if you're new to tools:

Concealer brush This makes it easy to apply concealer on hard-to-reach areas like the inner corner of your eye and along the lash line. You can also use this brush to spot-apply cover-up on blemishes.

Blush brush The wide, rounded shape and angled sides of this brush apply the perfect amount of powder blush on the apples of cheeks. It gives you a seamless and natural-looking flush.

Eyebrow brush Use the angled head of this brush to apply eye shadow to brows, shaping and filling them in for a natural look.

Eye-shadow brush The small, fluffy bristles of this brush pick up the just the right amount of eye shadow for your lower lid.

Eyeliner brush This is the easiest way to draw a line that's just right—not too thick or thin. This brush can be used dry with eye shadow, or damp for more definition and long-lasting liner.

Think of these as intermediate brushes. They're nice additions as you get more comfortable with your routine:

Foundation brush Ideal for creating a polished look with full coverage. This brush can be used with liquid and cream foundation formulas.

Powder brush The tapered head of this brush covers all the contours of your face, making it easy to dust on loose powder for an even, flawless finish.

Bronzer brush It's quick and easy to fake a sun-kissed glow with this broad brush. Use it to apply a seamless, streak-free dusting of bronzing powder.

Eye-shader brush This wide brush, which is shaped to cover the entire eye area, makes it quick and easy to apply light eye-shadow base.

Lip brush The small, firm bristles of this tapered brush make it easier to apply darker lip colors with precision. After lining lips, use this brush to soften and blend lip pencil lines.

Brow-groomer brush Use this toothbrush-style brush to comb brows into place for a polished look.

CARING FOR YOUR BRUSHES

With proper care, a good set of brushes can last you a lifetime. Clean your brushes regularly, at least every two to three months (more often if they become dirty or tough to use). Use a gentle soap like baby soap or baby shampoo to remove makeup and residue. Start by dipping the tip of the brush head in lukewarm water. Squeeze a small amount of soap in your palm, then wipe the wet brush in your hand to pick up the soap. Gently massage soap through the bristles. To rinse, swirl the brush tip in water. Pat the bristles dry with a towel and shape them as needed. Lay the brush over a counter edge to dry.

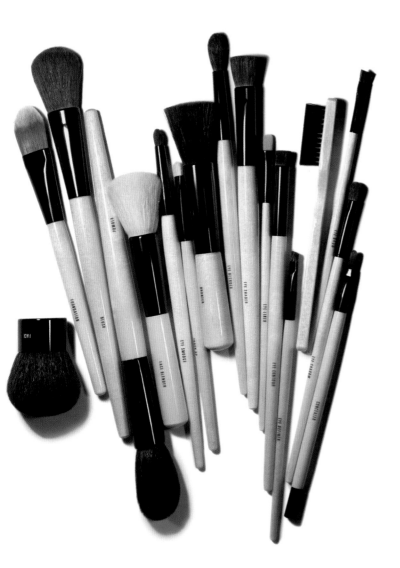

TOOLS OF THE TRADE

In addition to your brushes, be sure to include these other tools in your makeup kit for a flawless face.

MAKEUP SPONGE

Ideal for applying and blending foundation and cream makeup formulas.

EYELASH CURLER

A good choice if you have lashes that stick straight down. Choose a metal curler with rubber pads.

TWEEZERS

Great for quick brow cleanups. Look for tweezers with angled tips that can grab even the finest hairs.

How to Achieve Flawless Skin

The Basics

Some women are born with flawless skin. Other women, myself included, need to put in a little work to achieve the look. The good news is that getting gorgeous skin is easier than you might imagine. What's the secret? It's all about the right concealer, foundation, and powder.

Concealer

If I had to pick one product that most dramatically improves a woman's appearance, it would be under-eye concealer because of the way it magically brightens up the face. Concealer is the best way to lighten dark circles (and look rested—even when you're not!). Choose a yellow-toned concealer that is one to two shades lighter than your foundation. Pass on concealer that is too light, is too pink or white, or is chalky or greasy.

Use a small-headed brush with firm bristles to apply a generous amount of concealer under the eye, along the lash line and innermost corner of the eye. Gently tap the concealer with the pad of your index finger to blend it in. Try to apply as little pressure as possible. Tugging and rubbing will simply wipe concealer off. If you still see darkness, apply a second layer of concealer.

Avoid midday creasing by locking the concealer in place with loose powder. Use a velour puff or small powder brush to apply the powder. For the most natural look, use white powder if you have very light skin and yellow-toned powder if you have light, medium, or dark skin.

Foundation

Foundation is my trick to achieving a smooth and even complexion. As a makeup artist, I've found that yellow-toned foundation looks the most natural on all skin tones. To find your perfect match, swipe a few shades on the side of your face and check your reflection in natural light. The shade that disappears is the right one. If you have to apply foundation on your neck to make it match your face, you're using the wrong shade. It's a good idea to have two shades of foundation—one for the winter months and a slightly darker one for the summer when skin color tends to warm up.

Use your fingers or a makeup sponge to spot-apply foundation where skin needs to be evened out, especially around the nose and mouth where there's redness. For full, allover coverage, use a foundation brush to apply and blend foundation.

Foundation formulas range from low-maintenance tinted moisturizers to moisturizing liquid and cream foundations with more coverage. Here's a look at what the different formulas have to offer:

Tinted moisturizers and tinted balms combine the benefits of a face cream with the skin-evening properties of a foundation. They're a good choice for normal and normal-to-dry skin that needs minimal coverage.

Liquid and cream foundations are available in both moisturizing and oil-free formulas. They are easy to blend and can go from medium to full coverage depending on how much you apply. If you go for liquid, be sure to shake the bottle first to make sure heavier parts haven't settled to the bottom.

Stick foundation is one of my favorite formulas because it's portable and quick and easy to apply. A good choice for normal skin, this travel-friendly formula won't ever spill and can also be used to cover blemishes and scars.

Compact foundation, with its powder formulation, is best for oily skin. To avoid looking cakey, look for one that's not too powdery. Many compacts come with different sponges that allow you to control the amount of coverage you get.

Powder

To give foundation staying power and take away shine, finish off with a dusting of powder. I believe pale, yellow-toned powder is the most flattering on all skin tones. A big beauty myth is that translucent powder is invisible. I find that it actually makes skin look pasty and ashy. The same holds for purple, pink, or green powders designed to "correct" color—they don't look natural, so stay away from them. Look for a powder with a silky, lighter-than-air texture. I use loose powder at home and pressed powder when I travel, since it's more portable. Use a velour puff to apply the powder and dust off any excess with a powder brush. Apply a fair amount of powder if skin is oily. Dust it just around the forehead, nose, and chin if skin feels dry.

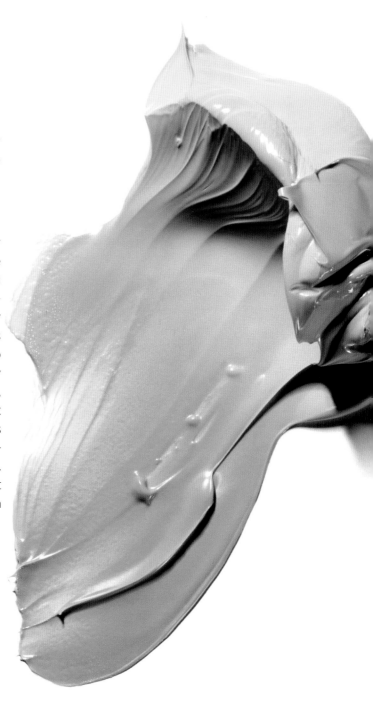

Step by Step
to Simple Beauty

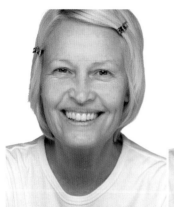

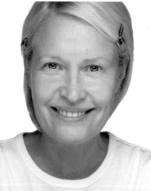

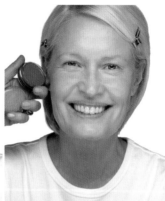

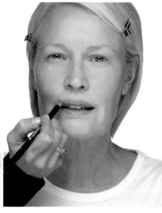

GUNILLA WITHOUT MAKEUP
A few easy steps and the right products were all Gunilla needed to bring out her natural beauty.

CONCEALER / FOUNDATION / POWDER
I used yellow-toned concealer to cover the pink under Gunilla's eyes, and evened out her complexion with tinted moisturizing balm and a touch of powder.

BLUSH
To brighten up Gunilla's face, I applied creamy pink blush to the apples of her cheeks.

LIP COLOR / LIP LINER
Gunilla has a lot of pink in her lips, so I played that up with pink gloss and liner.

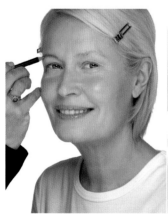

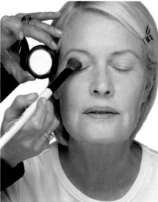

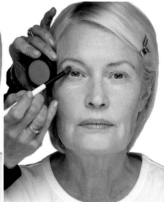

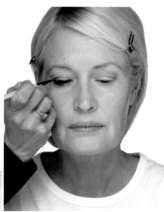

BROWS
I filled in sparse areas in Gunilla's brows and created a natural-looking shape with a soft brow pencil.

SHADOW 1
To brighten up Gunilla's eyes I used white shadow all over.

SHADOW 2
I dusted grey shadow on her lower lid.

LINER & MASCARA
I applied cobalt blue gel liner on Gunilla's upper lash line to lift and open up her eyes. Two coats of black mascara was all Gunilla needed to enhance her lashes.

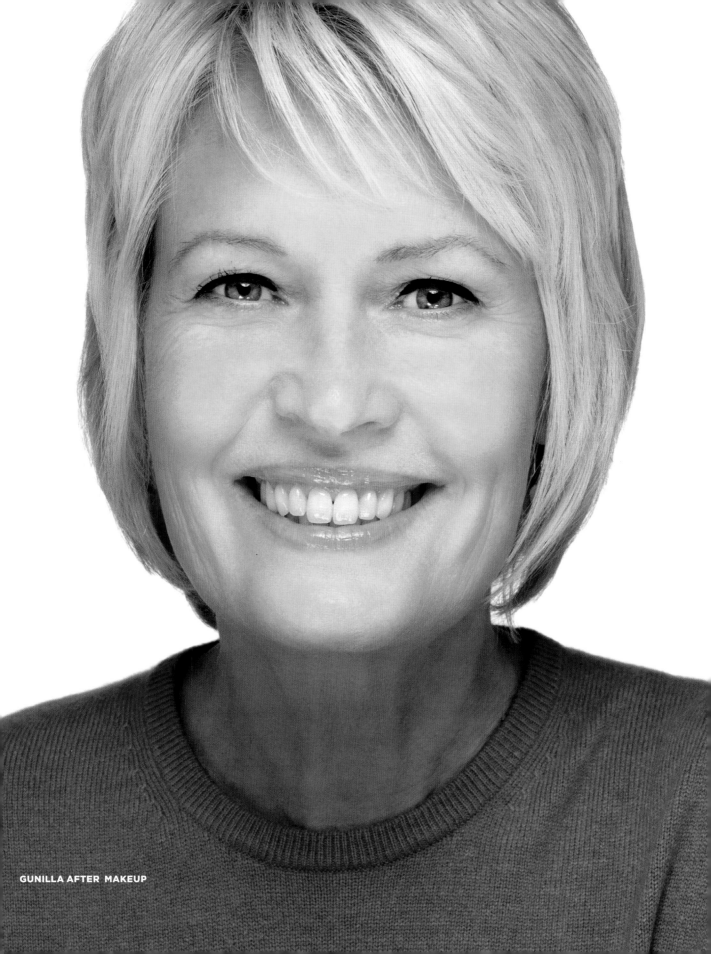

GUNILLA AFTER MAKEUP

Beauty Issue
Extreme Under-Eye Darkness

Under-eye circles are the bane of most women I know. They're the result of a combination of factors. Some of the factors are beyond our control—like the aging process (the skin around the eye area becomes thinner, so superficial blood vessels show through even more), genetics, and allergies. Other factors that are within our control include sleep, stress, smoking, and how we take care of ourselves.

Beauty Rx

There are no products on the market that actually lighten under-eye darkness. At best, eye cream can hydrate the eye area and give it a fresher look. It's crucial to find one that hydrates lightly to ensure that your under-eye concealer goes on smoothly. A richer, deeper treatment formulated with shea butter and beeswax works best overnight to keep skin hydrated in the morning.

I've found that the best way to brighten extremely dark under-eye circles (circles that have a greenish or purplish tinge to them) is to start with a pink- or peach-toned corrector, then layer on the yellow-toned concealer. The pink or peach shade may work alone sometimes, but mostly you'll need to layer it. For problem dark circles, keep the focus on the upper part of your eyes. Many women with extreme under-eye darkness also have dark eyelids, so lighten the area with light (white or bone) shadow. Don't line the lower lash line or apply mascara to lower lashes. A pop of bright pastel pink or peach blush on the apples of your cheeks will also steer your eye away from the dark circles.

A BOBBI POINTER: THE RIGHT CONCEALER

Sometimes you need to change your concealer color to a lighter shade or another tone because of factors like a change in seasons, hormonal changes, lack of sleep, or stress. There are times when what works for me in the morning doesn't work for me late in the afternoon. It's worth it to have an arsenal of concealer colors—it'll do more for you than an extra lipstick. Spend wisely.

A BOBBI POINTER: EYE OPENER

Applying concealer on the hollow sides of the nose (the spot next to the eye socket) will open up your eyes and make them look bright and awake.

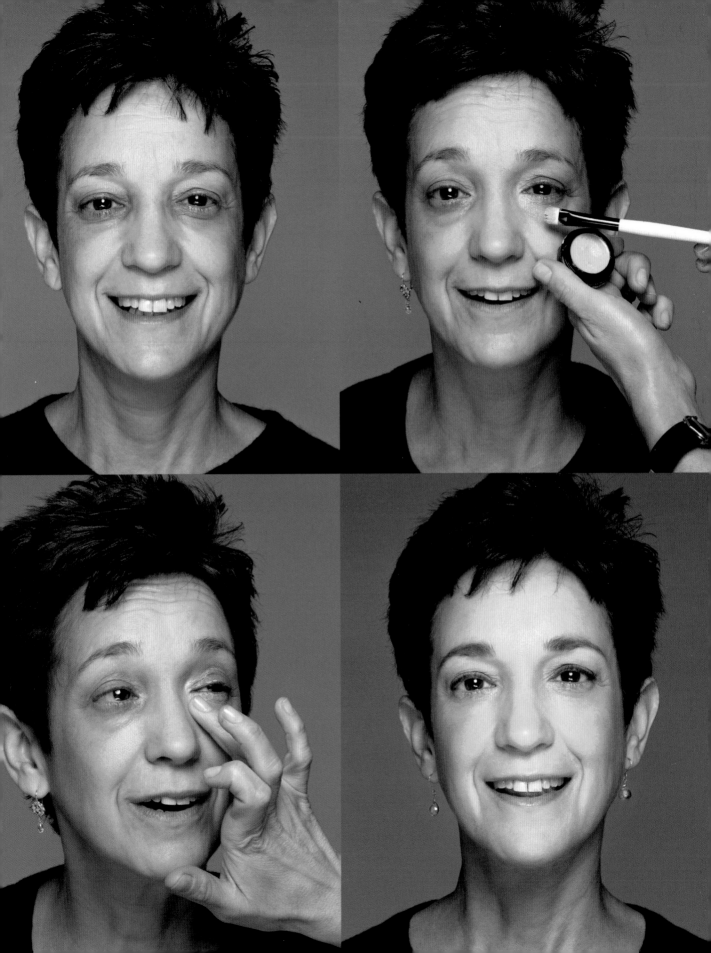

Beauty Issues
Fine Lines, Wrinkles, and Loss of Elasticity

Fine Lines and Wrinkles

Fine lines and wrinkles are an unavoidable part of getting older and they happen to all of us. There are some mornings when I look in the mirror and see lines that I swear weren't there the night before! Instead of freaking out, I give my skin back the moisture it's lost by drinking plenty of water and reaching for my arsenal of creams and oils.

Beauty Rx

The truth is that there is no cream on the market that gets rid of wrinkles, but you can greatly reduce their appearance by using the right moisturizers in the right combination. Depending on how dry your skin is, you may use one or all of the following: a face oil, a hydrating cream, and a soothing balm. You want to gauge how much your face needs at that particular moment.

If your skin feels really tight, start with an emollient face oil. Look for one with natural essential oils like sesame, sweet almond, and olive oil—these help restore the natural levels of lipids in dry skin. If it feels like you have an oil slick on your face, use your hands to blend the oil in. Next, apply a hydrating cream that's formulated with deeply moisturizing ingredients like squalene or petrolatum. Warm the cream in the palms of your hands, then gently pat the cream into your skin. Wait a few minutes, and if the skin still feels dry, apply more cream. When I'm really dry, I finish with a soothing balm patted just on the driest parts of my face (look for one that contains shea butter and beeswax).

Now that your skin is well hydrated, you're ready for makeup. I like tinted moisturizing balms and moisture-rich foundations, which soften lines and wrinkles rather than settle into them. Check the label on the makeup for ingredients like sodium hyaluronate, which bonds moisture to the skin, and petrolatum, which creates a creamy consistency. I find color is equally important here. Make sure the foundation is the exact color of your skin. Otherwise no matter how great the formula is, it won't look good. Make sure the face is evenly covered, well hydrated, and soft before you continue with color.

Loss of Elasticity

Loss of elasticity is the result of a decrease in the protein elastin in your skin. As its name suggests, elastin gives skin its elasticity and allows it to stretch and snap back into place. Other factors like yo-yo dieting, sun damage, and smoking all contribute to the skin's loss of elasticity.

Beauty Rx

I've seen improvements in my skin after using either a retinoid cream or a topical cream containing growth factors. Retinoids stimulate collagen production to help give skin a firmer, more toned look. Creams like Retin-A Micro and Renova both contain retinoids. TNS Recovery Complex, which contains growth factors, is a good choice if you have sensitive skin. But beware, it is expensive and has a very sour smell. (For more information on solutions available at your dermatologist's office, see Chapter 2.)

When it comes to makeup, the same cream-based makeup formulas that work so well on skin with fine lines and wrinkles work with elasticity issues too. Rather than trying to cover things up with too much makeup (the truth is, you can't disguise loss of elasticity), I believe in using makeup to divert attention away from the problem. Try darker eyeliner and a pop of brighter blush on the apples of your cheeks—both will give your face a lift.

Beauty Issues
Blemishes and Scars

Blemishes

As much as I hate to say it, blemishes aren't just a bane of our adolescence. Many women going through perimenopause and menopause complain about blemishes, and this is a side effect of the changing balance between androgen and estrogen. Rather than pick at the blemish (you'll risk infection and scarring), treat it with a topical retinoid and use some makeup to downplay it.

Beauty Rx

Never use concealer to cover blemishes; concealer is designed to be lighter than your skin tone, so it will actually draw attention to your blemish. A creamy, medium-weight cover-up or stick foundation is the best way to cover a blemish. Liquid formulas will be too sheer and won't offer enough coverage. Choose a shade that's the same color as your skin. To check, swipe the cover-up or stick foundation on the side of your face. If the swipe disappears into your skin, it's the right shade.

Use a concealer brush to spot-apply the cover-up or stick foundation just on the blemish. Pat with your index finger to blend. Then set the cover-up or stick foundation with sheer face powder applied with a velour puff or small powder brush. If you still see the blemish, repeat this process, layering cover-up/stick foundation and powder.

Scars

I love scars because I think they communicate character. Every scar is unique to the woman who has it—and that, to me, is beautiful. If you choose to cover your scar, you should know that you won't be able to conceal it 100 percent. However, there are certain products that you can use to make your scar less noticeable.

Beauty Rx

The best way to cover scars is with stick foundation or a dense, long-lasting concealer like CoverMark (a good choice if your scar is very prominent). Regardless of which product you choose, be sure to use a shade that matches your skin exactly.

Use a concealer brush to paint the stick foundation or concealer directly onto the scar. You may need to warm the product in the palm of your hand before applying it. Apply a little at a time and add more if needed. After you've covered the scar, use a velour puff to seal the stick foundation or concealer with a skin-tone-correct shade of face powder.

Beauty Issue
Uneven Texture

Some women complain that their skin doesn't look smooth. As we age, skin may change in texture and look slightly coarser than it did when we were in our twenties and thirties.

Beauty Rx

The good news is that you can make skin look smoother using the right foundation. After priming your skin with moisturizer, even it out with a whipped foundation in a shade that matches your skin exactly. Test the foundation by swiping it on the side of your face. Don't test it on your hand or your arm—your face is seldom if ever the same color as the rest of your body. (If the foundation disappears into your skin, it's the perfect shade.)

Whipped foundation, which comes in both moisturizing and oil-free versions, is very similar in consistency to pudding. This formula works well on textured skin because it acts like putty, filling in uneven spots. To keep skin natural looking, make sure the foundation blends down to a thin layer of coverage. If your skin is on the oily side, finish with a dusting of face powder on your forehead, nose, and chin (apply the powder with a powder puff, or for a more sheer finish, use a powder brush). The powder will not only keep the foundation in place but also help give your skin a smoother appearance.

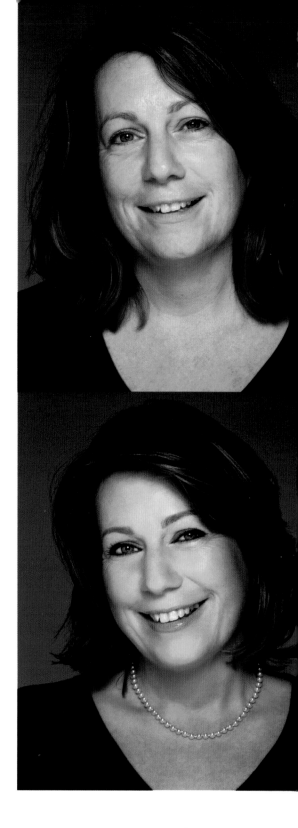

Beauty Issue
Uneven Skin Tone

This is a common problem faced by women in their forties and fifties—your skin is still smooth, but it's blotchy and uneven in color. You may have some redness around the nose and discoloration due to sun exposure and hormonal changes.

Beauty Rx

The best way to even out your skin tone is with a tinted moisturizer or foundation. For the most natural look, make sure the product you're using matches your complexion and is yellow-based. The majority of women, from the fairest to darkest complexions, have yellow undertones in their skin, so a pink-based product will look unnatural and "masky." The tinted moisturizer or foundation shouldn't change the color of your face; it should even out your skin tone. Apply the tinted moisturizer or foundation to even out skin, especially around the nose, mouth, and side of the face, where there's often redness.

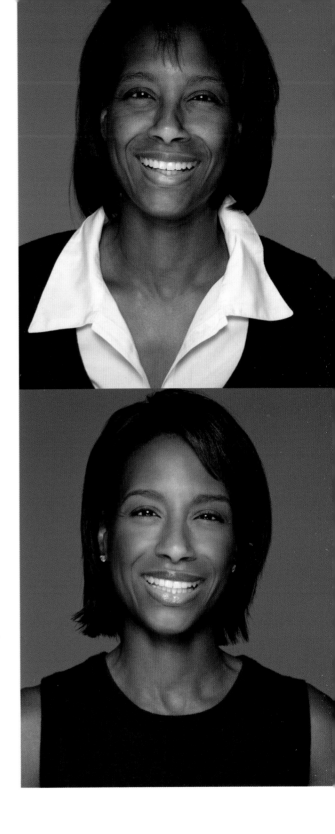

Beauty Issue
Ruddy Skin and Rosacea

Ruddiness is often a precursor to rosacea (a skin condition that causes redness and pimple-like outbreaks), so take steps now to care for your skin before any major flare-ups occur. Whenever a woman comes to me for advice on dealing with ruddiness, the first thing I do is ask her about her skincare regimen. I find that many women use cleansers and scrubs that are much too harsh and actually irritate their skin.

Beauty Rx

If you're a big outdoorsperson, be sure to protect your face extra well with a sunblock of at least SPF 30 (I see a lot of skiers who have ruddy skin because they hit the slopes barefaced). Try not to aggravate your skin with strong face scrubs or masks, and skip any products that contain alpha hydroxy acids. Use a soapless cleanser and extra-gentle facial moisturizer (face oil works too). If the redness persists, ask your dermatologist about treating your rosacea with a topical solution. Metronidazole, which is available in cream, lotion, and gel form, helps kill the bacteria that cause rosacea.

A yellow-toned tinted moisturizer or foundation is the best way to tone down ruddiness. Don't bother with the green or purple correctors you see in some stores—you'll just end up looking like you have green or purple color on your face. Using a makeup sponge or brush, gently apply the tinted moisturizer or foundation all over the face. Next, spot-cover any areas where you still see redness with a touch-up brush and stick foundation. If you still see red in your cheeks, skip blush and simply finish your face with a light dusting of bronzing powder. The brown tones in the bronzer will help counteract the redness. To ensure a seamless look between your face and neck, be sure to apply bronzer on your neck as well.

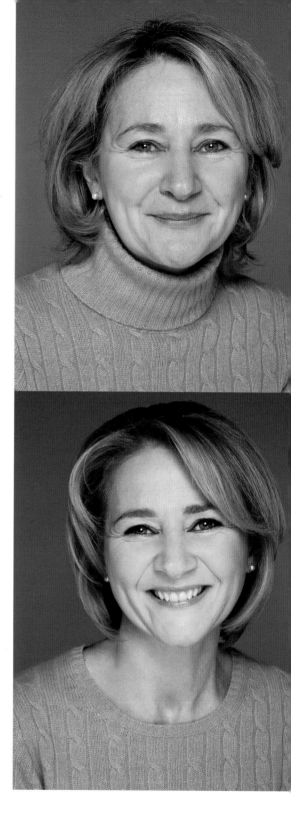

Beauty Issue
Brown Spots

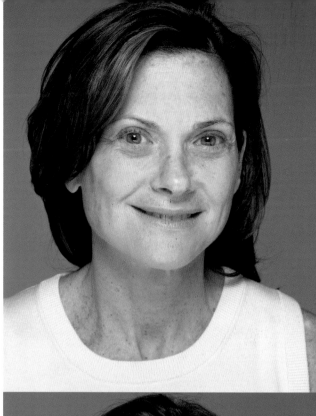

Brown spots are the result of too much sun exposure and often genetics. Many women think these spots are an inevitable part of aging and simply attempt to cover them with lots of heavy makeup. But unless you are heavily freckled, you don't have to live with brown spots. By removing them, you look younger and fresher.

As I confessed in Chapter 2, I was a sun worshipper when I was younger (I used baby oil, iodine, and homemade reflectors), and I know a lot of damage has already been done. But it's never too late to start protecting your skin. So if you don't already, you should wear sunblock on a daily basis. Throw on a baseball cap if you plan on being outdoors for an extended period of time.

Beauty Rx

There are many over-the-counter and prescription-only bleaching products that claim to lighten dark spots. I've tried a few of the options and I've been underwhelmed by the results. In my opinion, nothing works as well in removing brown spots as laser resurfacing performed by a dermatologist (for more information on laser resurfacing, see Chapter 2). I've been extremely happy with the results of laser resurfacing on my skin.

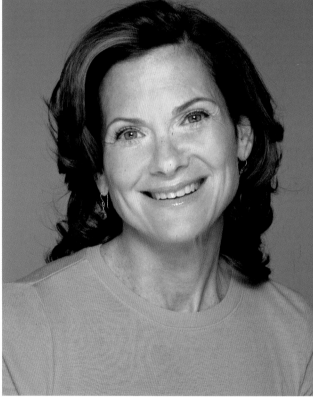

If you're not ready to try a laser, or if you still have faint spots even after the treatment, you can use makeup to make the spots close in color to the rest of your face. Use concealer approximately two to three shades lighter than your skin. Using a concealer brush, apply concealer just on the spot. Then gently pat the concealer with your fingers to blend it in. Follow with foundation applied all over the face. To avoid rubbing the concealer off, use a light hand when smoothing on the foundation. Set the concealer and foundation with face powder that matches your complexion.

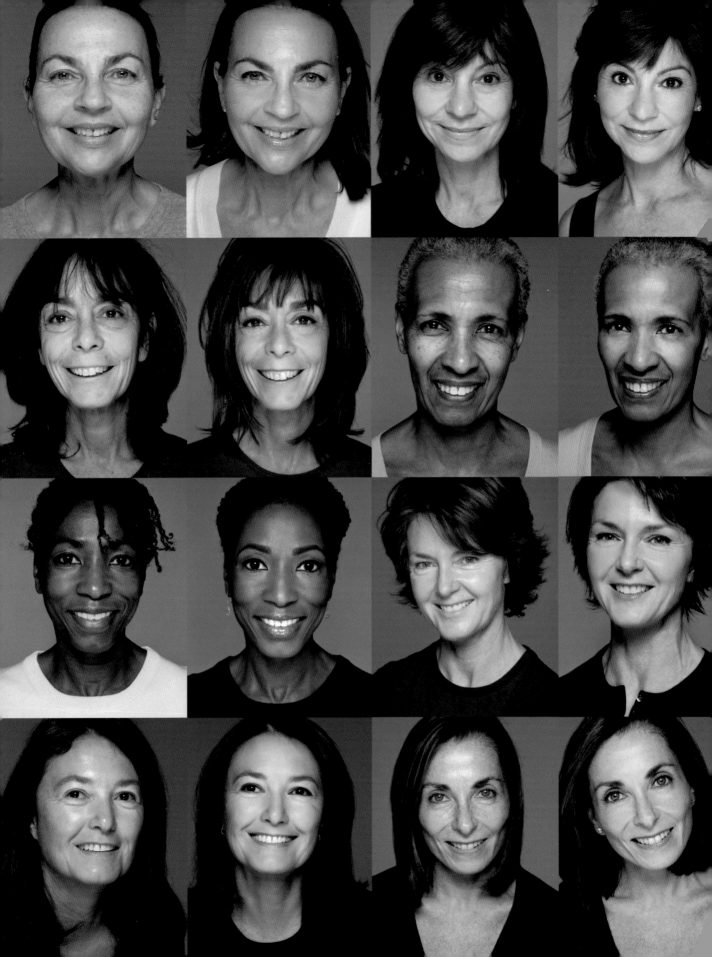

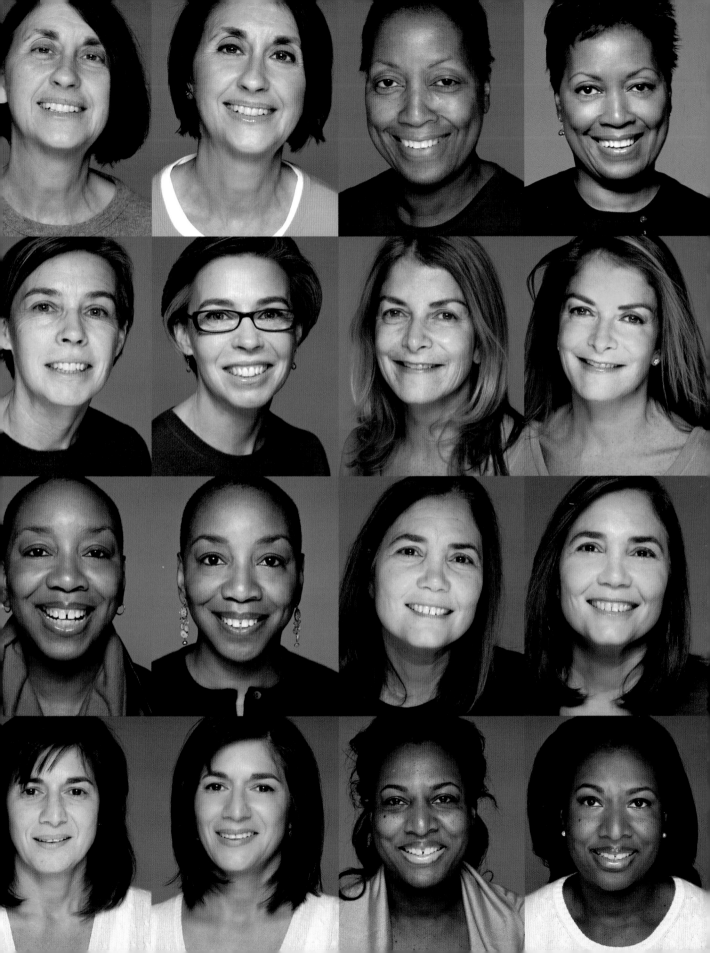

How to Get a Healthy Sun-kissed Glow

I've always loved the healthy, outdoorsy look. When everyone was doing neon-bright makeup in the 1980s and early 1990s, I was into creating natural-looking faces that featured bronzed skin and flushed cheeks. It's still my favorite look today.

Bronzers

Bronzers come in a few different formulations. If your skin is normal to oily, select a powder bronzer and apply it with a short, fluffy brush. Another option is a cream bronzer, which is ideal for dry skin and can be applied with fingers or a sponge. For the most natural look, apply the bronzer where the sun naturally hits your face—your forehead, cheeks, nose, and chin. Be sure to dust your neck and chest if you're wearing a bare top.

The most natural-looking bronzers have predominantly brown tones (with a bit of red) to them. Avoid bronzers that are orange-toned or frosted because they look artificial on any complexion. Most companies offer light, medium, and dark shades. Pick your shade based on how you tan naturally. For example, if you turn a medium golden brown in the sun, a medium bronzer is your best bet. The bronzer should blend easily and warm up your face. If the color looks too orange or obvious, try one shade lighter.

For a sun-kissed look that lasts a few days, try self-tanner. Self-tanners have improved a lot in recent years and I've gotten great, natural-looking results. But before slathering yourself in self-tanner, do a patch test on the inside of your arm to make sure you're not allergic to the formula. To ensure that color develops evenly, be sure to exfoliate any rough patches before you apply the tanner. When applying self-tanner to your face, spread a thin layer to start. If you want to go darker, you can always wait until the color develops and do another application. Avoid your eyes and make sure to get your ears and neck so that there aren't any obvious lines. Be sure to wash your hands thoroughly after applying self-tanner, and allow enough time for it to absorb before getting dressed or going to bed. If you wake up the next day to mistakes like too-dark color or obvious streaks, you can fade them with a gentle exfoliant and lots of moisturizer.

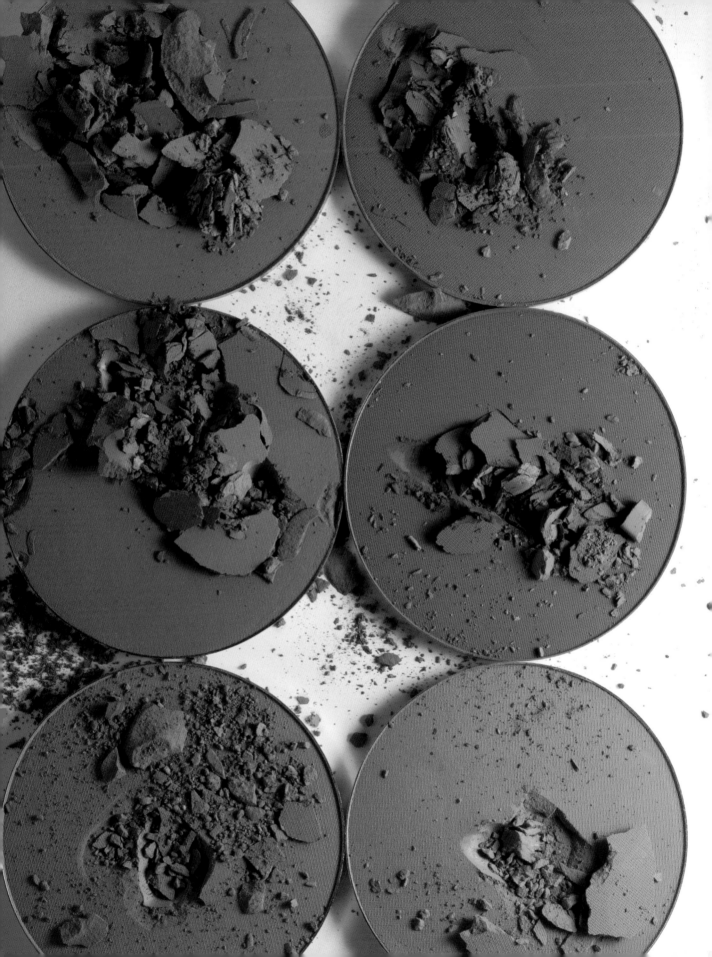

Blush

I am obsessed with blush because I think it makes everyone look prettier, not to mention the fact that it's an instant face brightener. A woman should have at least two blush colors: a natural one and a pop of color. Your natural shade of blush should look like your cheeks when you're naturally flushed (or after you've exercised). Your pop of color should be brighter and clearer (less muted)—for example, pink, coral, rose, or plum. (See photo, opposite page.)

Blush comes in a few different formulas:

Powder blush is the easiest formula to work with. Powder blends well and works on the majority of skin types. Mistakes like too-strong color can be corrected easily and blended with a clean powder puff.

If you have dry skin or like a dewy look, choose a cream blush. The emollients in this formula do double-duty, moisturizing skin and helping color glide on effortlessly. It gives skin a nice glow, but isn't particularly long-lasting. Avoid cream blush if you have rough skin or breakouts.

Cheek tints/gels offer sheer color, but they take some trial and error to blend just right. This is a good choice for anyone who has very oily skin. But if you layer on too much, you run the risk of looking splotchy.

FIND YOUR MOST FLATTERING SHADE OF BLUSH USING THIS GUIDE:

COMPLEXION	BLUSH SHADE
Porcelain	*Pale pink or pastel apricot*
Fair	*Sandy Pink*
Medium	*Tawny brownish pink*
Tan	*Deep browish rose*
Olive	*Plum, golden brown, or deep rose*
Dark	*Dark or deep bronze or deep red*

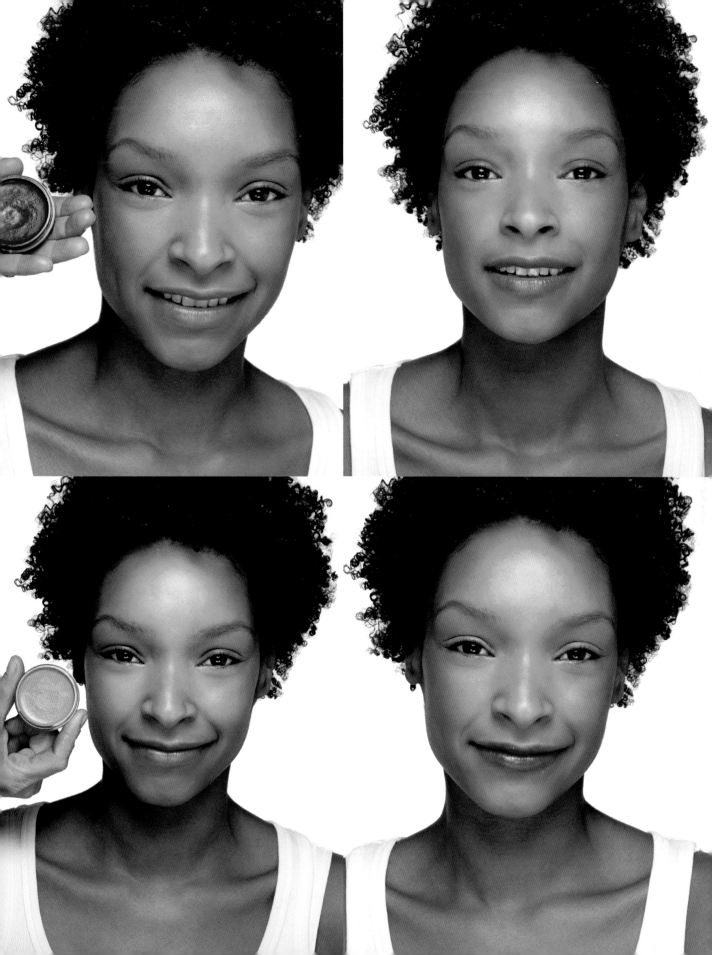

Beauty Issue
Dull, Sallow-Looking Skin

Many women complain of dull, "blah-looking" skin, especially in the winter months. Bare skin will look faded and washed out (the result of slower skin cell turnover) and cheeks won't have that just-pinched look you see in children. Instead of throwing your arms up in defeat, counteract dull skin by exfoliating and adding color back with makeup. Women are always amazed when I show them how easy it is to re-create a youthful glow.

Beauty Rx

When choosing a scrub, go for one made specifically for the face. Scrubs made for the body are far too abrasive for the face and will end up irritating your skin. Glycolics, which are part of the alpha hydroxy acid family, work by speeding up the process through which skin sloughs off the outermost layer of dead skin cells to reveal fresher skin. (You can find more skincare tips about glycolics in Chapter 2.)

After your scrub reveals fresh skin, use a self-tanner or bronzer to neutralize the sallow, yellow-green tones in your face. Next, reach for a bright blush to give your cheeks a "pop" of color. If you're not into bronzer, use two shades of blush to get your glow. Start with a neutral shade of blush that looks like your cheeks when they're naturally flushed or when you exercise. If the color is hard to blend, it's either too dark or too bright. Smile and apply blush to the apple of the cheek, then blend up and back toward the hairline. To make the color look like it belongs on the skin, blend it down as well. Finish with a pop of brighter blush on the apples of your cheeks.

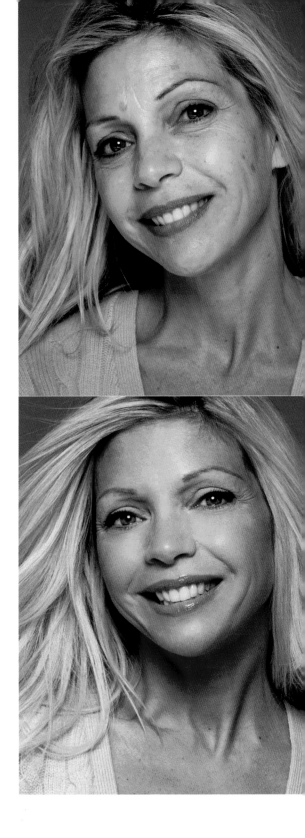

A BOBBI POINTER: BRIGHTEN UP

Every single woman I know, no matter what her age, wants her skin to look bright and luminous. It's a quality that you see in children, teenagers, even women in their twenties and thirties. The bad news is that we lose this natural glow as we get older. The good news is that you can brighten up with makeup. Here's how:

• Tinted balm evens skin out and gives it an instant glow.

• Warm moisturizing balm in the palms of your hands, then pat the balm over your blush.

• After applying blush, dust a shimmering powder high on the cheekbone.

• When you're finished putting on your makeup, gently apply face oil on top.

• Wear cream blush instead of powder blush.

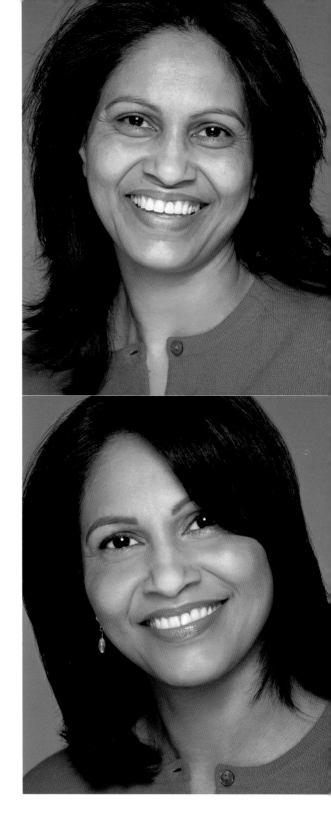

How to Color Lips

Choosing a great lipstick color is more about your personal style than hard rules. For a no-fail natural-looking lipstick, you should take into account the coloring of your skin, your hair, and your lips (this is why a lipstick color that looks great on your friend's lips doesn't always look so good on you). The most flattering shade will be one to two tones darker than your lips. If you are fair-skinned, choose shades of beige, pale pink, and light coral. Medium skin tones look great in brown-based shades of rose, mauve, and berry. Pick deep plum, chocolate, and red if you have dark skin. When choosing your lip color, think about how it's going to balance your eye makeup. A light, neutral lip is the perfect contrast to strong eye makeup. A bright or deep lip is a good complement to simple eye makeup. (And all the rules are off for some women who are just plain red, pale, or dark lipstick lovers.)

Start with clean, smooth lips. If you have dry flakes, gently exfoliate them with a damp washcloth. Moisturize your lips with lip balm or eye cream. Neutral colors and sheer formulas can be applied directly from the tube. Use a lip brush to apply darker and brighter colors that require precise application. For natural-looking definition and to keep color from feathering, line lips with lip pencil after applying lip color. Soften and blend any harsh edges with a lip brush.

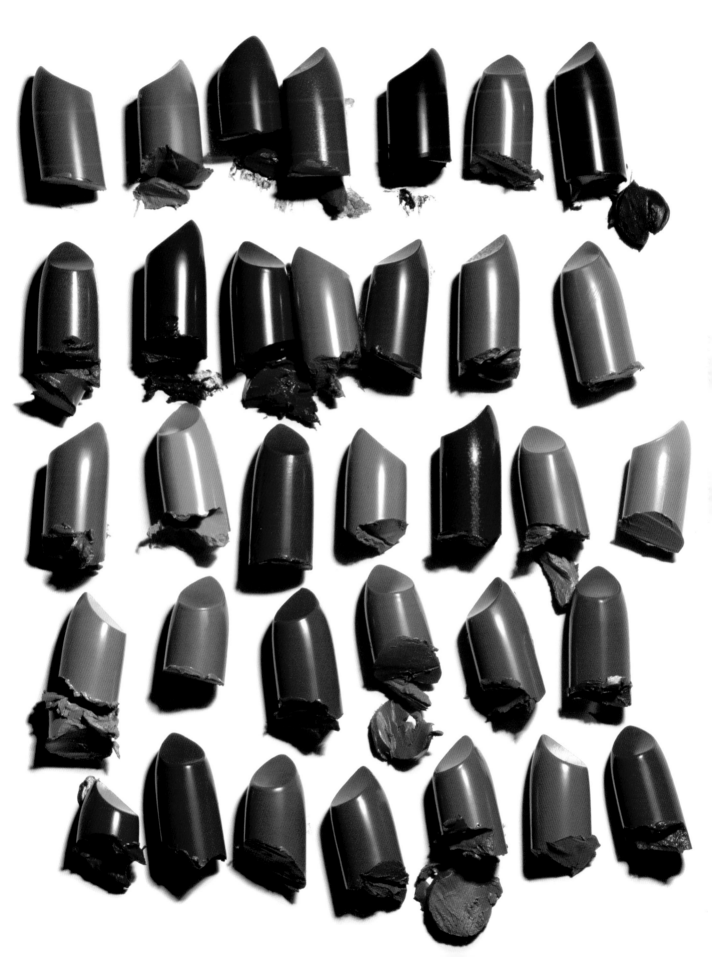

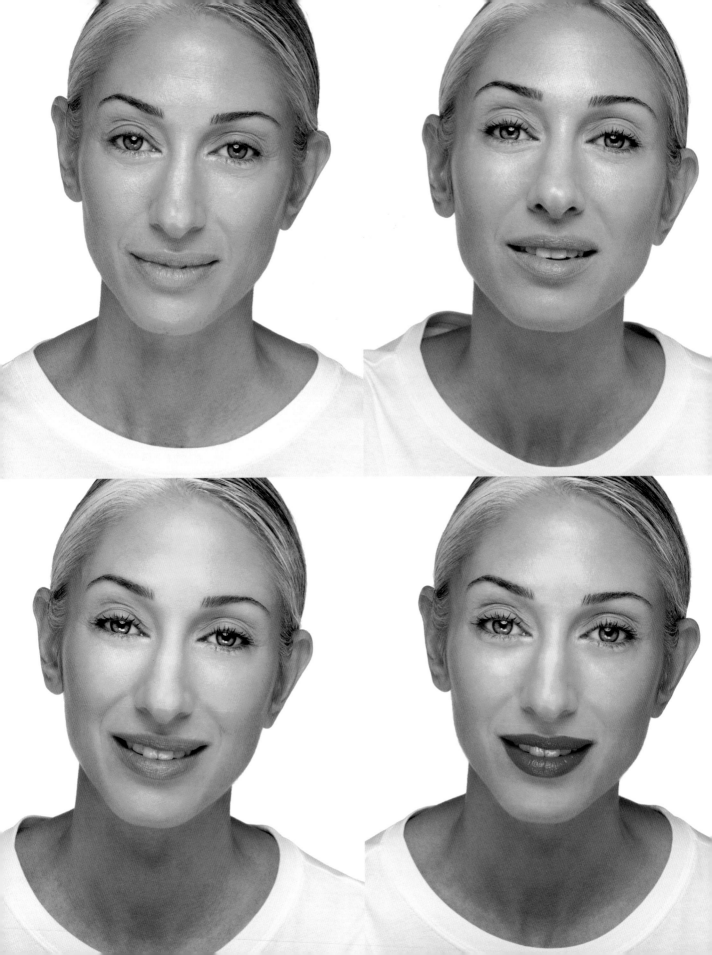

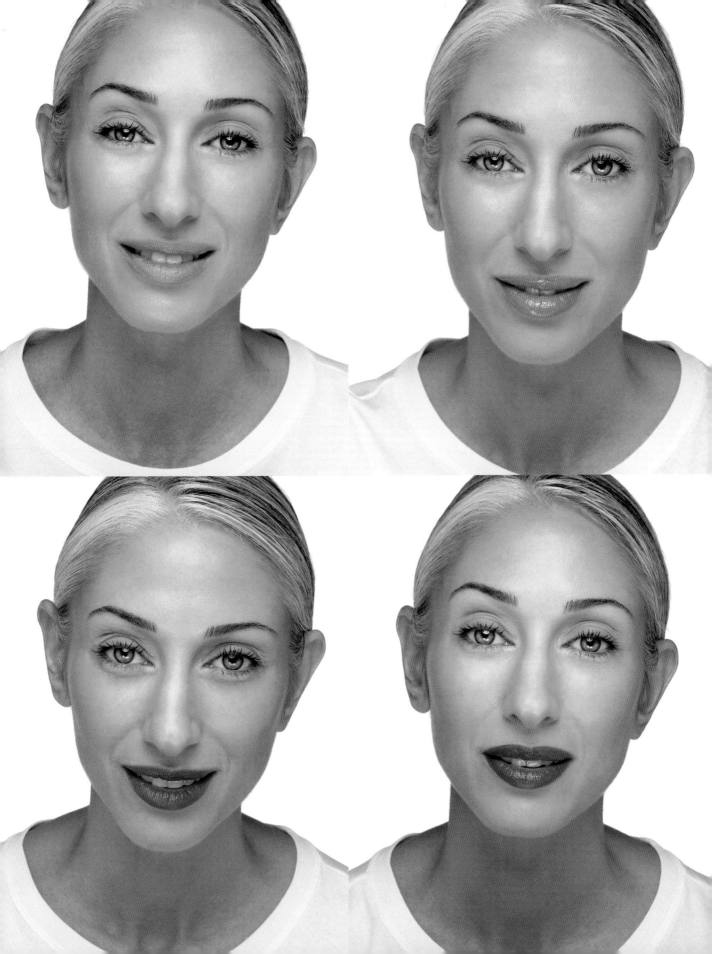

Beauty Issues
Thin Lips, Loss of Definition, and Lines Around the Mouth

Thin Lips

One of the complaints I often hear from women when they hit their forties and beyond is that their lips no longer have that plump, "pouty" look. Some thinning of the lips is the result of a decrease in collagen production. And some women, desperate for the fuller lips of their youth, resort to treatments like fillers. I think it looks fake, lumpy, and horrible. Small lips—your lips!—are better than fake lips.

Beauty Rx

Stick to light-to-medium lip color shades and avoid dark shades, which have a minimizing effect and make thin lips look even thinner. Choose shiny glosses and creamy lipstick formulas—they impart a sheen that helps create the illusion of fullness. Finally, line the very outer edge of your lips using a pencil one shade deeper than your lipstick (don't draw outside your mouth, as this will only look like you've lined outside your lips). And don't waste your money on balms, lip glosses, or lipsticks that claim to plump up lips—they don't work.

Loss of Definition

I usually wear little or no makeup. However, over the last few years I've become more diligent about wearing makeup because it gives my face back some of the definition that it's lost. When women ask me how to define lips, I always suggest a lipstick and pencil the color of your own lips.

Beauty Rx

To give lips definition, I like to line the lips with a neutral lip pencil after applying lipstick or gloss. For the most natural look, I use a slightly darker, lip-toned lip pencil (be careful—if you use an overly dark shade of pencil you'll end up with that obvious ring-around-the-lips look). If you can see the pencil after you've applied it, use a lip brush to soften and blend the harsh edges.

Lines Around the Mouth

Given all the negative effects that smoking has on our health and our looks, I'm still surprised when I see people lighting up. Smoking is one of the main causes of lines around the mouth (the result of repeatedly pursing the lips). Genetics and sun damage factor in too.

Beauty Rx

You can lessen the look of the lines around your mouth with prescription-only creams containing retinoids or growth factors—both help stimulate collagen production. (For more on these solutions, turn to Chapter 2.)

Before applying any color to your lips, plump and soften the lines with a hydrating cream, and make sure your lips are moist (using a rich lip balm or eye cream works well too). I don't suggest overly glossy lip formulas because they have a tendency to creep off lips and into lines. Instead, try lip pencil paired with a creamy matte lipstick. Line and fill in your lips with the pencil, then apply a coat of the lipstick (it will truly be budge-proof). If you want a bit of shine, you can top the lipstick with a bit of gloss (it won't run because it will adhere to the lipstick).

Beauty Issues
Loss of Color and Uneven Lip Color

Loss of Color

Lips with a natural cherry-stained color are a sign of youth. As we get older our lip color fades, but this beauty problem is an easy one to fix. It's time to update your makeup bag with some fresh hues.

Beauty Rx

Now more than ever, the right shade of lipstick or gloss will make a huge difference in your appearance. Toss out the beiges and browns that you loved when you were younger—now they'll just make your lips look even duller. A great trick here is to find a lipstick that is the shade of your lips and blends into the bottom lip without turning orange or brown. To add color and vibrancy back to lips, choose medium-toned hues of pink, rose, berry, or apricot.

Some women have the opposite problem of lips that darken with age—the trick here is to find a lipstick that lightens and brightens without looking gray. My aunt Alice used pale pink lipstick to lighten her naturally brownish blue lips. Choose between beige, pale pink, or pale peach lipsticks. I sometimes apply foundation on bare lips to help lighten them before applying lipstick. But be careful—this can look ashy and make your lipstick cakey.

Uneven Lip Color

Many women don't naturally have a uniform color to their lips—often, one lip is darker than the other, particularly among darker-skinned women. Rather than making lips one color, play up the difference—it's a beautiful thing!

Beauty Rx

You can use either a light shade to play up the light part of your lip or a dark shade to enhance the deeper part of your lip. If you're really bothered by the difference in color, you can even out your lips by using a sheer dark lipstick as a base on the lighter lip. Then apply your regular lipstick or gloss on both top and bottom lips. Finish with lip pencil in a shade that matches the darkest part of the lip and blend well.

**A BOBBI POINTER:
THE PERFECT LIP COLOR**

◆

Make your own lip stain.
Mix lip balm and your favorite color
lip pencil directly on your lips.
Rub your lips together,
then blend the color into your lips
with your fingers.

How to Groom
Your Brows

Well-groomed brows frame your face and give it a more polished look. It's amazing how plucking and filling in the brows can lift and open up the eyes. Here's how to get perfect arches:

Pluck any stray hairs between the brows. The inner corner of the brow should line up with the inner corner of the eye. Tweeze hairs growing below the brow. Pull hairs in the direction they are growing, in one quick motion. To enhance the natural arch of the brow, tweeze hairs just below the arch. Clean up stray hairs above the outer corners of the brows.

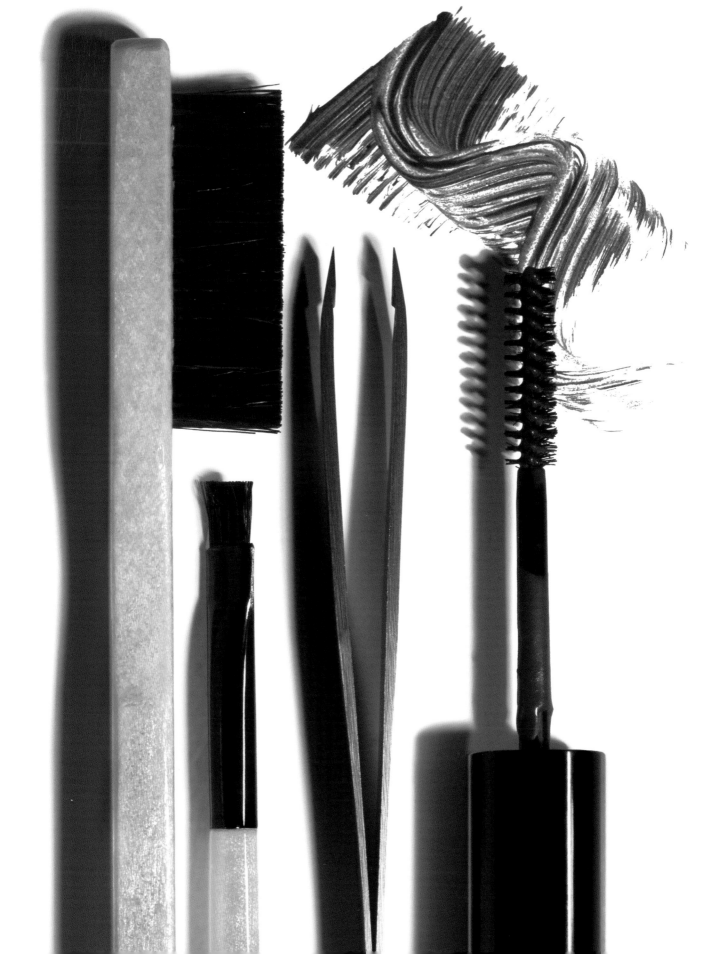

Beauty Issue
Sparse Brows

I've always loved eyebrows. I began to appreciate mine as a teenager when I saw Ali MacGraw in the movie *Love Story* because it was the first time I saw a beautiful woman with strong brows. I think brows add strength to a woman's face and give it a more polished look. They also draw attention to and bring power to the eyes. If your brows are sparse from years of overplucking, illness, or medication, you can give them a boost with makeup.

Beauty Rx

Use a soft eyebrow pencil to fill in sparse areas or holes in the brow. For the most natural look, draw in short, hairlike lines. Once you've filled in your brows, soften the lines by layering powder shadow (it should be the same color as the eyebrow pencil and hair) on top. Apply the shadow using an eyebrow brush with bristles that are stiff and angled at the tip. If the brow color looks too strong, tone it down by pressing loose face powder onto your brows with a powder puff. Finish with a coat of brow grooming gel to keep individual brow hairs in place. How do you know what eye pencil or eye shadow shade is best for your brows? The right brow color should complement your hair color.

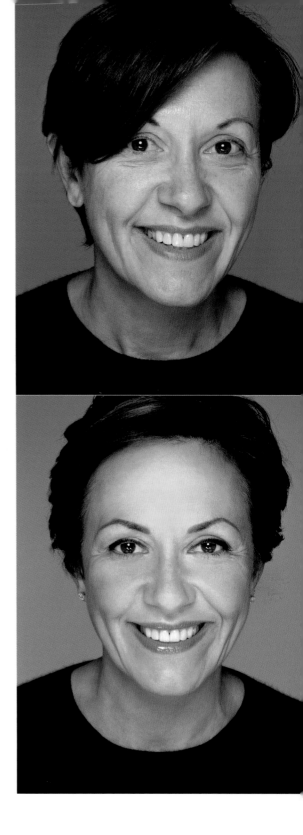

Hair Color	Brow Color
Pale blonde	Light ash blonde
Medium to dark blonde	Ash blonde to sable
Light to medium brown	Sable to mahogany
Medium to dark brown	Mahogany to reddish brown
Black	Mahogany to smoke (never black)
Light red	Taupe or camel
Medium red	Taupe to reddish brown
Dark red	Reddish brown
Slate	Mahogany or dark gray
Light gray	Slate or gray
White	Gray or taupe

How to Get Standout Eyes

When choosing eye makeup, take into consideration your natural coloring and personal style. For some women, a neutral eye shadow and a coat of mascara are more than enough. And then there are other women who feel their best with full eye makeup: base color, lid color, contour, highlighter, liner, and mascara.

Eye shadow

You have a few choices when it comes to eye shadow:

I love powder shadow because it is versatile and easy to work with. Choose from soft matte (an all-around flattering option) or shimmery (find a formula that's more sheer than frosted). Leave the glittery shadows to the teens. Many powder shadows are formulated to be used dry or damp, which allows you to adjust the intensity of the color.

If you have especially dry eyelids, cream shadow is a good choice. Plus, it's incredibly portable and you don't need a separate brush to apply it. The downside is that some formulas tend to crease, so pass on it if you have less-than-smooth eyelids.

The longest-lasting shadow formula is cream-to-powder shadow. It's ideal if you have a lot of naturally occurring oil in your eyelids and looks best on smooth skin. To avoid a crepey effect, smooth cream-to-powder shadow on bare lids and don't layer it with other shadow formulas.

Eyeliner

To make eyes really stand out, line them. Here are your options for lining eyes:

Powder shadow is my go-to for lining eyes because it's easy to work with and very versatile (depending on how you apply it, you can create a clean, sharp line or a soft, diffused line). Use an eyeliner brush that's thin and flat with straight or slightly angled bristles. To prevent dark specks of shadow from falling under the eyes when you line, lightly blow or tap on the brush to get rid of excess shadow. My other trick is to dampen the brush before I dip it into the shadow—in addition to ensuring that the shadow stays on the brush, this also makes the shadow last longer.

Eye pencils are a popular option because they're relatively mistake-proof. They're a good choice if you don't want to fuss around with a separate makeup brush. The downside is that their wax-based formula makes them prone to smearing. If you can't part with your pencil, consider layering powder shadow over it to make it longer-lasting.

For the most dramatic effect, go for liquid or gel liner. The waterproof, long-lasting formula makes this a good choice if you're prone to tearing or want your liner to last from day to night.

As I mentioned earlier, I don't believe in a one-size-fits-all approach for applying eye makeup. However, here is my basic step-by-step for creating a classic eye. You can use it as a starting point and adjust it depending on the occasion or how much time you have.

1. Choose a light, medium, and dark eye shadow shade. **2.** After sweeping the light shade all over the lid, use an eye shadow brush to dust the medium shade on the lower lid. **3.** For added definition, apply a deeper shade on the outer corner of the eye. **4.** Finish by lining eyes with gel liner or a dark shade of eye shadow. You can line just the upper lash line or both upper and lower lash lines. If you choose to line eyes all around, make sure top and bottom liner meet at the outer corner of the eye.

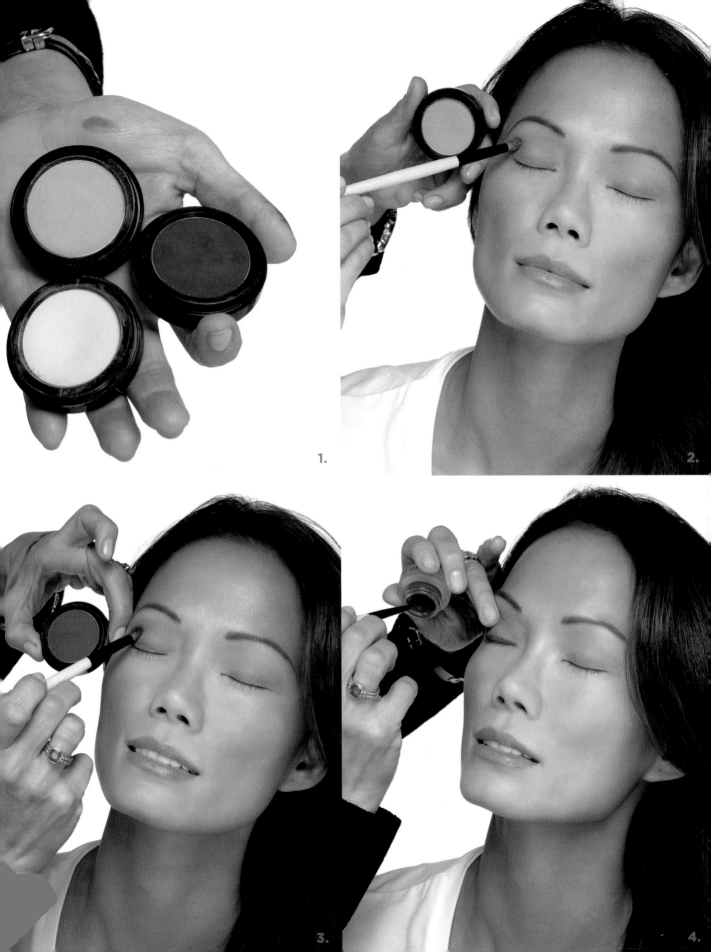

1.

2.

3.

4.

Mascara

Many women I know would never dream of leaving the house without mascara on. And with good reason—it's an easy way to dress up your eyes. Mascara comes in a range of formulas that offer different looks and benefits. Here's a look at the most popular formulas available today:

Thickening mascara Pigments, waxes, and film formers in the formula build up individual lashes to create a denser look—making it ideal if you have a sparse lash line. Thickening formulas usually come with brush wands that have tightly packed bristles to allow for thicker application.

Lengthening mascara Lengthening mascaras add length to short lashes with special filament-type fillers—lashes are enhanced, but still natural-looking. The formula is thinner in consistency than the thickening variety, so it goes on in sheer coats. The thin, widely spaced bristles on the brush wand of lengthening mascaras define lashes without adding bulk.

Waterproof mascara This long-lasting formula contains special pigments that resist moisture. It's a good choice if you want mascara that will stay on through a workout or if you're prone to tearing. Strong polymers in the formula can dry out lashes, so you might not want to wear it seven days a week. To get waterproof mascara off, you'll need an oil-based makeup remover.

I think that darkest black mascara looks great on most everyone. Choose brown mascara if you want a more natural look. Pass on trendy colors like blue, plum, and hunter. Before applying mascara, blot the end of the brush on tissue to get rid of excess mascara. Don't pump the wand in the tube because this will push air into the mascara and cause it to dry out. Holding the mascara wand parallel to the floor, work from the base to the tip of the lashes. Roll the wand as you go to separate lashes and avoid clumps.

Always apply mascara to upper lashes from underneath; brushing mascara over the top will weigh the lashes down. If you choose to apply mascara on lower lashes, use a lighter hand than you did on upper lashes. Apply one to two coats for a subtle look and two to three coats for a more dramatic effect.

A BOBBI POINTER: CURLING CUES

I recommend curling lashes if you have lashes that stick straight out or point downward. Use a lash curler that's wide enough to cover the entire lash line and make sure that the rubber pads are in place properly (otherwise the metal edge of the curler will break your lashes). Always curl mascara-free lashes; curling lashes after applying mascara makes them more prone to breakage. For the best curl, start crimping at the base of the lashes and hold the curler for a few seconds as you lift up.

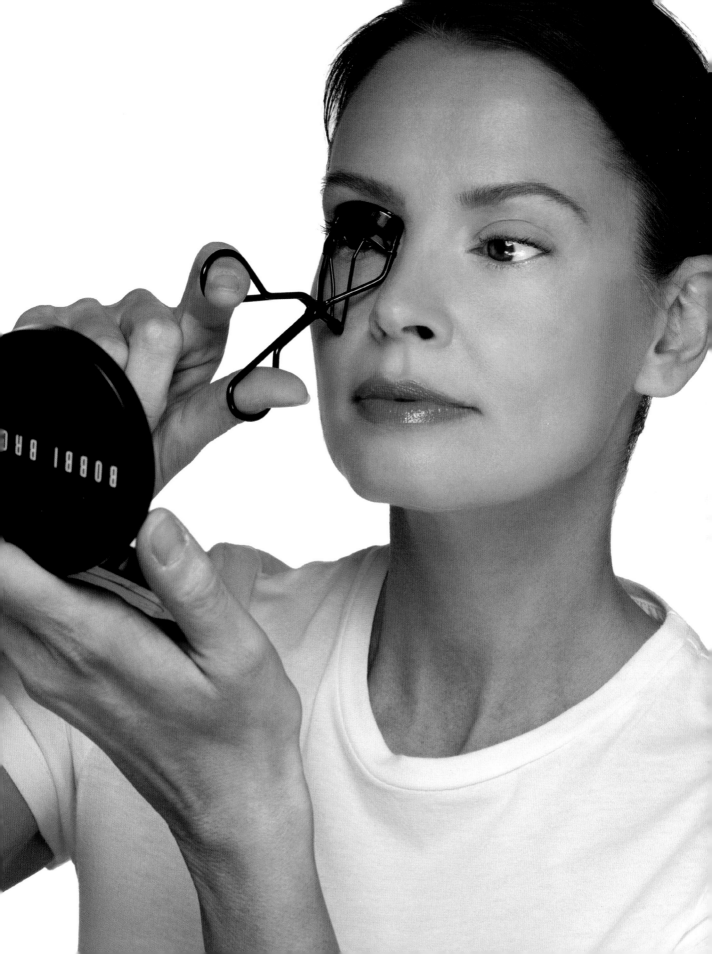

Beauty Issues
Loss of Eye Definition and Crepey Eyelids

Loss of Definition

I was in my forties when I really began to notice changes around my eyes. Up until that point, I had always kept my eye makeup pretty minimal. But I realized that I now had to use liner daily in order to give my eyes back the definition they no longer had.

Beauty Rx

Eyeliner is the most effective way to add definition to eyes. Choose a dark liner shade like mahogany, navy, forest green, or black. Start on the upper lid and be sure to apply liner as close to the base of lashes as possible. Work from the inner corner of the eye to the outer corner. After lining your upper lash line, look straight into the mirror to check your work. The liner should be thick enough to be visible when your eyes are wide open. If you want to, you can line the lower lash line as well; use the same liner color that you applied on the upper lash line, or go one shade lighter for a softer, yet still defined look. Make sure that both lines meet at the outer corner.

A deeper medium tone of shadow is optional for those of us who need extra definition. Apply the medium shade on the lower lid from the lash line to three-quarters of the way up. Two to three coats of a very black mascara will also do wonders to make eyes stand out.

Crepey Eyelids

Crepey skin around the eye area is the result of aging, too much sun exposure, and genetics. Get in the habit of wearing sunglasses when you're outdoors. And don't worry, there's help.

Beauty Rx

Before applying any eye makeup, press face powder (use a velour puff) on your lids to help create a smoother-looking surface. Don't apply foundation to lids—this will cause eye shadow to cake, exaggerating the crepeyness. Steer clear of shimmery eye shadow formulas, as they reflect light and draw attention to less-than-smooth lids. Cream shadow will work as long as the formula is not too greasy and not too drying. Your best bet is to pick soft matte shadows in light to medium tones of nude, brown, gray, and lavender.

A BOBBI POINTER: BLACK EYELINER

◆

Black liner is a big secret to gorgeous, sexy eyes—even for women who like the natural makeup look. Layer black liner on top of your normal liner (just on the upper lashline). Brush on two coats of black mascara and you'll see a real difference.

Beauty Issues
Droopy and Dark Eyelids

Droopy Eyelids

I've always found that "bedroom" eyes (which many women call "droopy eyes") are incredibly sexy—the actress Ellen Barkin comes to mind. But as we age, some of us have eyelids that go beyond bedroom eyes into the realm of just plain tired. I hate to admit this, but I have seen women who have had surgery to lessen the problem and look good. But I do believe that surgery is a last resort and makeup can do wonders to give your lids a lift.

Beauty Rx

A properly shaped brow can give your eyelids a more lifted look. Nature has already given you the best shape for your face—your job is simply to fine-tune it. Tweeze hairs between the brows and underneath the arch. Next, define your brows with a powder shadow applied with a brow brush (see the guide on page 79 to choose the best shadow color for your brows). Brush brow gel through brows to keep them in place.

Another lid-lifting trick is to line your eyes all around with a dark powder eye shadow applied with an eyeliner brush. The liner on the upper lash line should be thicker and stronger than it is on the lower lash line. To ensure this, line the upper lash line first. Then, line the lower lash line using the leftover shadow on the brush. Both lines should be thin at the inner corner of the eye and slightly thicker at the outer corner. Make sure the top and bottom lines meet at the outer corner of the eye and blend slightly upward to give eyes a lift. A very dark gel liner works great too.

If you're feeling ambitious or you're pretty comfortable with makeup, you can try contouring your eyes with a medium-deep shade of shadow like brown, slate, or mocha (the shade should blend easily). Starting at the upper outside corner of the eye, sweep the shadow in and down toward the crease of the eyelid. Next, sweep the shadow from the outside lower corner of the eye up to the crease (you're basically drawing a sideways V). The trick here is to layer a little color at a time (rather than blending, which can be hard and tricky). Highlighter applied on the brow bone (the area just below the arch of the brow) also helps draw attention up and away from the droopiness. After applying your eye makeup, rub your finger in white or bone eye shadow. Then gently pat the shadow on your brow bone. Finish with two coats of very black mascara to lift and define even more.

Dark Eyelids

I think it's a beautiful thing when a woman has a lot of color in her lids—I look at it as a natural eye shadow. The next time you look in the mirror, you might just find that your "problem" isn't so bad after all.

Beauty Rx

There are no skincare products for treating eyelid darkness. The good news is that you can easily lighten up the eyelid area using makeup. First, apply a loose yellow-toned powder on your lids. You can either press the powder on with a velour puff or dust it on with a wide eye-shadow brush. To further brighten the eyelid area, apply a light allover shade of soft matte eye shadow. Choose white if you're fair, bone if you have light to medium skin, and banana if you have darker skin. On the lower lid, try light shades like cream, pale pink, and peach. Avoid dark shades (they will make your eyes recede) and rosy or red-toned shades (they will make eyes look even more tired).

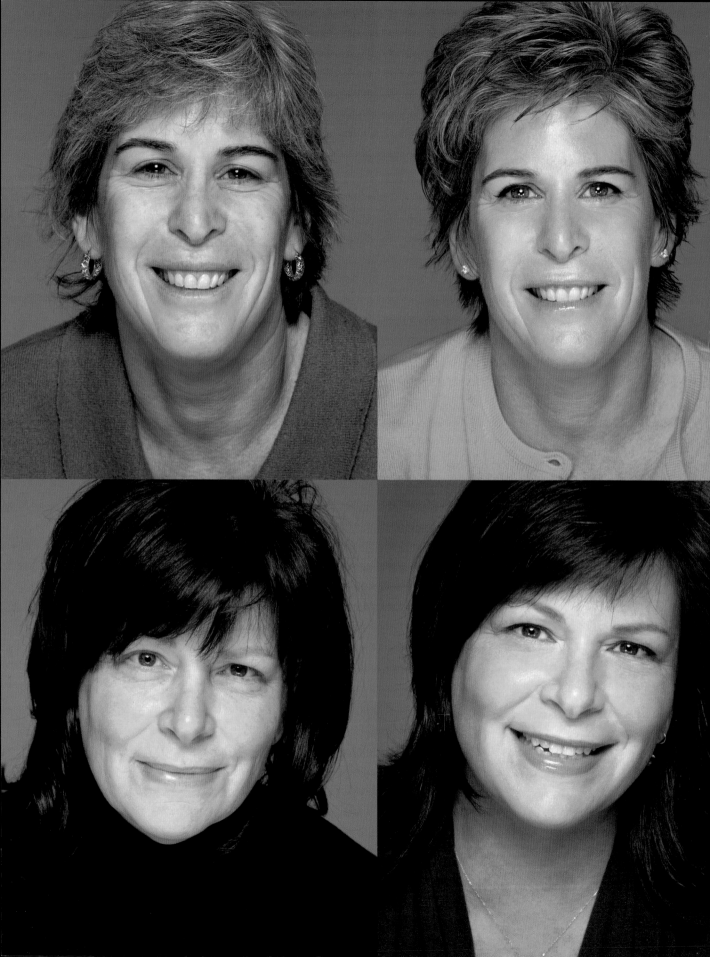

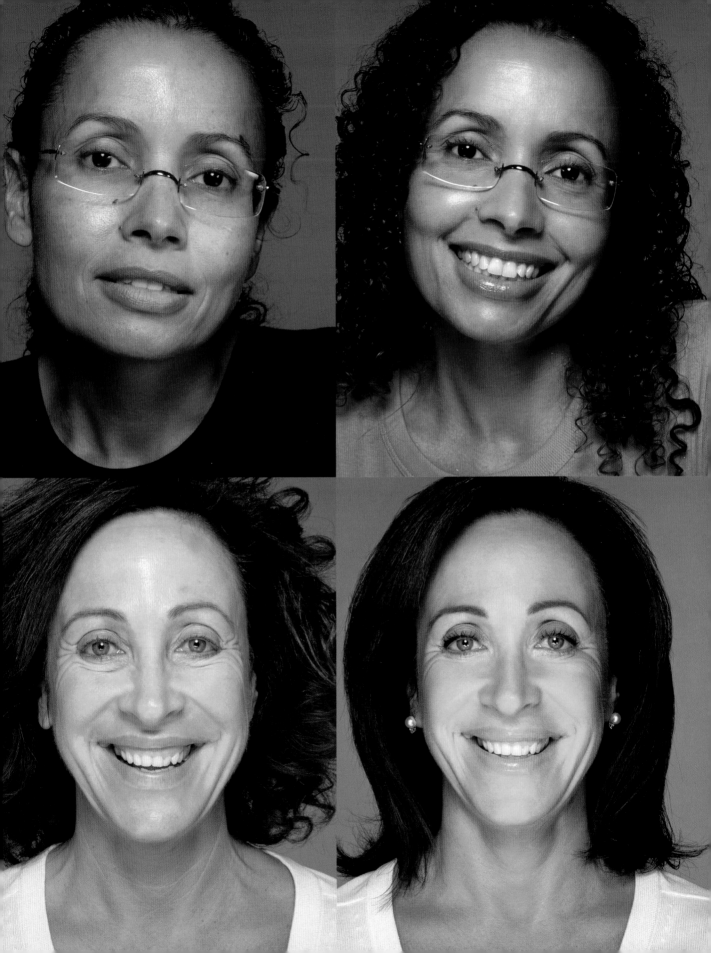

Beauty Issue
Skimpy or Nonexistent Lashes

Most women know the power of mascara—so it's no surprise that mascara is the number-one make-up product that women consistently buy over the course of their lives. That's why it can be disconcerting if your eyelashes start to become more sparse as a result of aging or illness. Overcompensating with more mascara just looks bad. The trick is to pair mascara with eyeliner.

Beauty Rx

Create the illusion of volume by applying two to three thin coats of very black mascara to lashes; layering coats is far more effective than applying one thick coat. Then, draw a smudged line along the length of the lash line. This will help create the look of thicker lashes.

A BOBBI POINTER: FAKING EYELASHES

If you've lost your lashes due to chemotherapy, create the illusion of hair by double-lining eyes. Using a dry eyeliner brush, apply dark powder eye shadow (dark brown, gray or charcoal) as close to the base of the lashes as possible; the line should be thick and smudgy. Repeat the process, this time with the brush slightly dampened. Use a stamping motion to draw a thinner line.

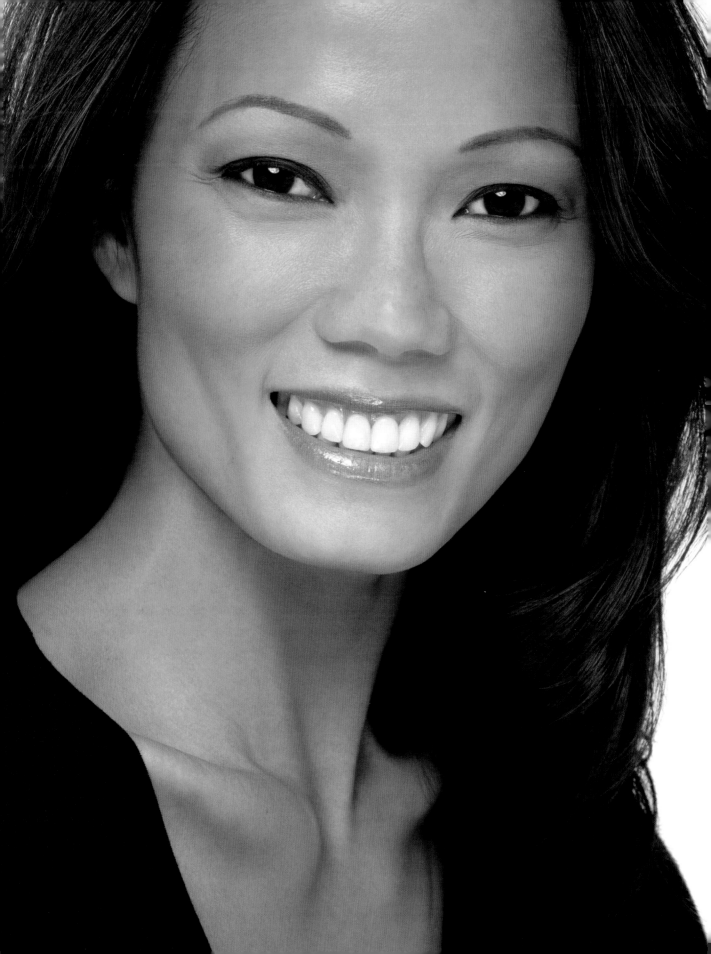

Perfectly Framed
Makeup Tips for Eyeglasses Wearers

Wearing glasses draws plenty of attention to your eyes, so it's best to keep your eye makeup simple. If you overdo your eye makeup, it will just clash with your frames and end up looking garish. Less is definitely more in this instance: line just the top lash line; dust a neutral, ashy shadow on the lower lid; and brush a thin coat of mascara on top lashes only. Save the bright and bold colors for your lips.

Eyeglass frames draw attention to the brows, so be sure to keep your arches well groomed. Pluck or trim any straggly hairs, and fill in holes in your brows with a brow pencil or powder shadow.

If your prescription makes your eyes look smaller, line your eyes—it's a surefire way to make them look bigger. Apply liner on both top and bottom lash lines to create a doe-eyed look. If your prescription makes your eyes look bigger, use a light hand when applying eye makeup and be sure to blend everything. The last thing you want your glasses to do is to magnify sloppy work!

P.S. When shopping for frames, look for neutral colors. I prefer brown, black, or clear plastic frames, or gold or silver wire frames. Brightly colored frames become dated very quickly.

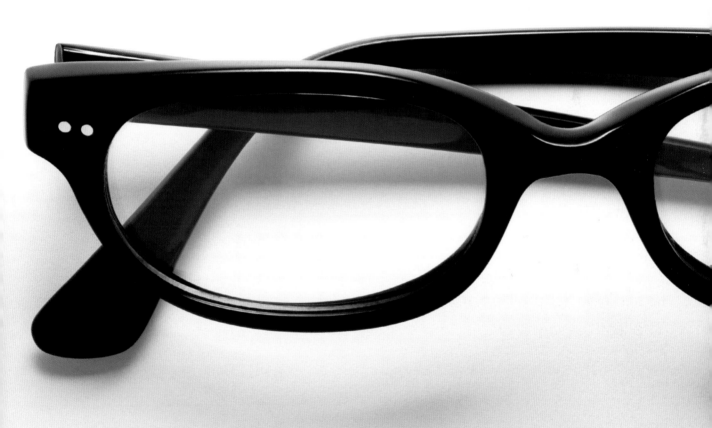

How to Pack the Perfect Makeup Kit

It's a good idea to have two different makeup kits—one that you keep at home and one that you carry with you for touch-ups during the day or when you're traveling.

At-Home Kit
Cleanser (face wash and eye makeup remover)
Eye cream
Moisturizer
Concealer
Foundation
Loose powder
Eye shadow (light, medium, and dark shades)
Mascara
Bronzer
Blush
Lipstick
Lip gloss
Lip liner
Makeup brushes (eyebrow, eye shadow, eyeliner, concealer, powder, blush, lip)
Tools (makeup sponges, velour puff, tweezers, eyelash curler)

On-the-Go Kit
Concealer
Stick foundation
Pressed powder (if you have oily skin)
Blush
Lipstick or lip gloss

BEAUTY RITUALS TO BEAT THE BLAHS

◆

Take relaxing baths. Sometimes you just need a few minutes of uninterrupted time to clear and rejuvenate your mind. Make it a point to pamper yourself at least once a week. Add soothing Epsom salts or skin-softening powdered milk to your bathwater—and watch all your worries soak away.

Dab perfume oil on your wrists, behind your ears, and on your collarbone. Scent is a powerful memory trigger, so choose a fragrance that makes you happy. Whenever I smell rose essential oil it reminds me of my childhood and spending time with my grandmother, who always wore rose perfume. Other essential oils remind me of great spa experiences that I've had.

Give yourself a manicure and/or pedicure—or better yet, go to the nail salon. This is the one thing that always makes me feel better instantly. Sheer and pale pink shades of polish are not only pretty, but also mistake-proof (there's no need to worry if you have a less than steady hand). Before applying polish, massage cuticles with olive oil that you've warmed in the microwave for a few seconds (wipe off oil on the nail bed before you polish).

───────

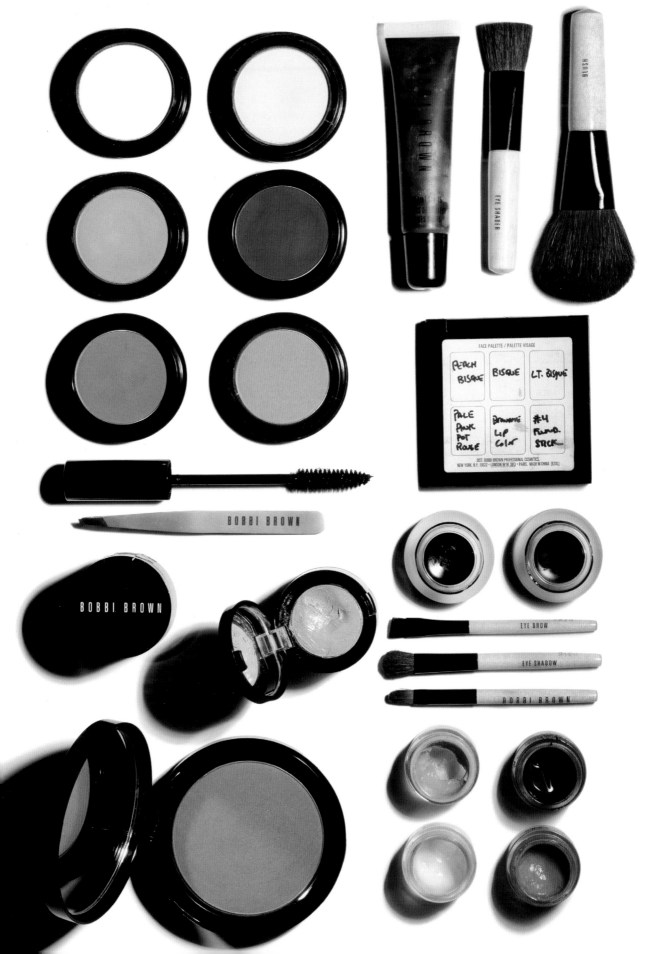

FACE PALETTE / PALETTE VISAGE

| PEACH BISQUE | BISQUE | LT. BISQUE |
| PALE PINK POT ROUGE | BROWNIE LIP COLOR | #4 FOUND. STICK |

DIST. BOBBI BROWN PROFESSIONAL COSMETICS.
NEW YORK, N.Y. 10022 • LONDON W1K 3BQ • PARIS. MADE IN CHINA [CZXL]

BLUSH

EYE SHADER

EYE BROW

EYE SHADOW

BOBBI BROWN

BOBBI BROWN

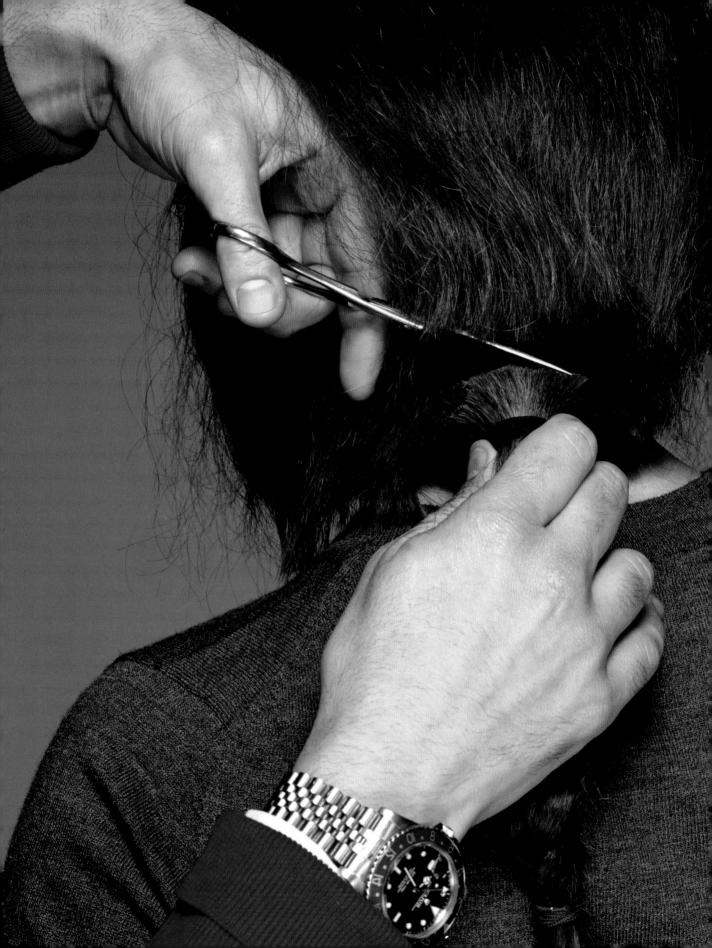

CHAPTER 4

YOUR CROWNING GLORY

How a Cut and Color Can Lift Your Look

I found my first white hair when I was twenty-five and I've been coloring my hair ever since. My salon visits were initially spaced every three to four months. Soon it became every six weeks. And I hate to admit it, but I now go every two to three weeks for a root touch-up. During one of my recent visits to the salon, I started chatting with some of the other women (there's not much else to do when you're waiting for the hair dye to process). We commiserated about the constant upkeep our hair requires and what a chore it is to keep it colored and cut to our liking. At one point, an older woman interrupted our complaining and wisely pointed out, "But, dears, at least we can do something...and look at the difference it makes." And she was so right.

I've tried many hairstyles over the years, including a layered shag, some bad perms, the sensible bob, and a pixie cut. I've learned (the hard way) that teased, overprocessed hair looks bad—no matter what your age. Get rid of that old-lady hairdo! Find the perfect simple cut. This is the time in your life when less is definitely more.

With the help of hairstylist Mario Diab, I've finally found the style that flatters me the most: a shoulder-length cut with a few soft layers. Some days I wear my hair wavy (I simply run some product through it and let it air-dry). Other days I like to blow-dry my hair straight. According to Mario, versatility is the key to a good cut. "Depending on how it's styled, a cut can look elegant and classic one day, then fun and modern another day," he says. I asked Mario to share his tips for making hair look its best. You'll find his expert advice and easy how-tos in this chapter.

All Your Hair Questions Answered

Bobbi—What do you suggest for someone who wants a modern, but not trendy, look? Mario—You can never go wrong with a layered bob—it always looks fresh. Or try a shoulder-length cut with long layers that are textured softly at the ends. If you want to go short, try a textured pixie cut (get shorter layers on top to create volume) à la Mia Farrow.

Bobbi—How should a woman decide what kind of haircut she should go for? Mario—More than anything, your haircut should be a reflection of your personal style. If you're easygoing and always on the go, choose a textured, short to medium cut. A good rule of thumb: the shorter your hair is, the less time you'll have to spend fussing with it. Allover layers are good because they give the cut a more casual look. This cut doesn't have to be overly styled to look good (just use some molding paste to separate the pieces). If your look is more classic and polished, go for a one-length bob or a medium-length cut with a few layers toward the front of the face. If your style is versatile and you like to change things up, you'll get a lot of mileage out of a shaggy medium-to-long cut with long bangs. During the day you can blow-dry the bangs and put the rest of your hair in a ponytail, or you can blow-dry your entire head straight and wear your hair down. For a more fun look at night, blow-dry the sections a layer at a time to play up the texture and give your cut more volume.

Bobbi—What's a good wash-and-go haircut? Mario—Your best bet is a short haircut with lots of texture. After towel-drying your hair, finger-style it using pomade. You can also try a layered bob haircut—to give it some shape and volume, hold your head upside down while blow-drying. Or you can try the never-fail ponytail.

Bobbi—Is there anything a woman can do to disguise thinning hair? Mario—Create the illusion of fullness with short-to-medium-length hair and allover layers. Add short textured pieces to help hold the layers. Consider using thickening shampoo and conditioner, as well as a thickening mousse or gel. These products are designed to build up on individual hair follicles to create the look of fuller hair.

Bobbi—How can you give your hair more volume? Mario—Ask your stylist for lots of layers on top and textured ends. When you style your hair, blow-dry in the opposite direction than the hair grows. For an added boost, try rollers. Apply volumizing mousse spray mainly on the roots, then put hair in rollers.

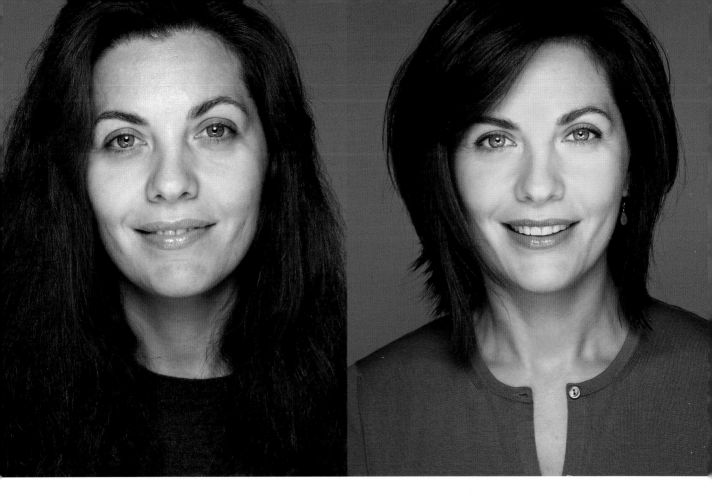

Bobbi—What's the best way to care for split ends?
Mario—Hair is a lot like a plant—it needs moisture to be healthy. Start by making sure you're drinking enough water. When you don't hydrate properly, your roots suck any moisture from the hair, causing it to dry and split. Use a moisturizing shampoo and deep conditioner at least twice a week for fifteen minutes at a time. Finally, ask your stylist to cut the split ends off (you'll need to cut at least half an inch). With proper care, the split ends shouldn't reoccur.

Bobbi—Do you suggest bangs to disguise obvious frown lines? Mario—Bangs are a great way to divert attention from forehead lines. Just make sure that your face looks good in bangs and that they don't overwhelm your face. A mistake many women make is getting heavy, blunt-cut bangs. Ask your stylist for a soft fringe and style your hair toward your face.

A BOBBI POINTER: DISGUISING THIN HAIR

You can also "color" in where your scalp shows through your hair using powder eye shadow (in a shade that matches your hair color) applied with a thick eye-shadow brush.

A Simple Guide to Hair Color

Bobbi—If a woman wants to change her hair color, how does she know what shade is right for her? Mario—Tear photos out of magazines and show them to your hairdresser. Sometimes what looks natural on one person looks over the top on another. Look at your natural coloring (the color of your eyes and complexion) to determine your tone. If you have blue, green, or hazel eyes and fair to light skin, you are a cool tone. If you have brown or black eyes and medium to dark skin, you are a warm tone. Cool tones look best with an ash or beige base (for single process). If you also want highlights, stick to the ash or beige color family. For warm tones, I suggest a medium to dark base (for single process) and honey or gold highlights.

Bobbi—Can a woman camouflage her grays without looking fake? Mario—Yes, but it becomes more complicated as the hair becomes grayer. Using one allover color will not only give you a harsh look, but also obvious roots. The best way to cover grays is with a combination of lowlights and highlights woven throughout the hair. Tip: If you're going from gray to brunette and don't want any red undertones (this is very common), ask your hairdresser to use ash or cool tones.

Bobbi—How does a woman go back to gray after coloring her hair for years? Mario—The transition to gray takes time and patience. The first step is to cut off the colored ends so that more of the gray root shows. Every six weeks, cut another quarter inch to half inch off. To minimize the contrast between new and old hair, use semipermanent lowlights where you part your hair.

Bobbi—What do you suggest to counteract the dulling and yellowing of gray hair? Mario—To neutralize the yellow, wash hair once to twice a week with a color-correcting violet shampoo. Counteract dullness with a clear hair-gloss treatment once a month; gloss treatments at salons are relatively inexpensive and the process only takes about fifteen minutes.

Bobbi—How often should a woman color her hair (root touch-ups and allover color)? Mario—If you are 100 percent gray, color your hair every three to four weeks. Go every five weeks if you are 50 percent gray. Roots need to be touched up every eight weeks. Allover color can be maintained with treatments every three months.

Bobbi—Should a woman color her hair at home or go to a salon? Mario—You can color your hair at home if you are making a subtle change in hair color. Leave drastic changes in color and highlighting to an expert.

Bobbi—What's your advice for coloring hair at home? Mario—Make sure you have all the necessary tools: gloves, a dark towel (if it gets stained with hair dye, it won't show), and a plastic cape (in a pinch, a trash bag will do). To protect skin from hair dye, apply a heavy cream or Vaseline along the hairline and on ears. After mixing dye, apply it immediately to hair (processing time starts the moment you mix the dye). Work dye through hair a small section at a time, making sure to saturate individual hairs from root to tip.

Bobbi—What can a woman do to make her color last longer? Mario—Avoid prolonged sun exposure and chlorinated swimming pool water—both fade color. Don't overwash your hair; shampooing two to three times a week is sufficient. Try a gentle shampoo formulated for color-treated hair or a color-infused shampoo to add depth and richness to your color.

QUICK FIXES FOR
WORKOUT HEAD

◆

I admit it. Every once in a while I skip a workout to avoid ruining a fresh blow-out (and many of my friends fess up to doing the same thing). And the truth is, I later regret it because I always feel better after breaking a sweat. I asked Mario for some tips on what I could do to maintain my blow-out while at the gym. Here are the secrets he shared with me (you'll never have to worry about workout head again!).

If you have long hair, put it into a high ponytail to keep your hair off your neck and back. When you tie your hair in a low ponytail, sweat from your head ends up accumulating at the ends.

To keep your bangs from getting limp and greasy, hold them off your face with a cotton headband. The headband will also double as a towel, absorbing any sweat along your hairline.

After your workout, dust baby powder onto a flat or round brush and run the brush through your hair. The talcum will soak up hair oils and perspiration. Get rid of any excess powder with a blow-dryer on its cold setting.

———————

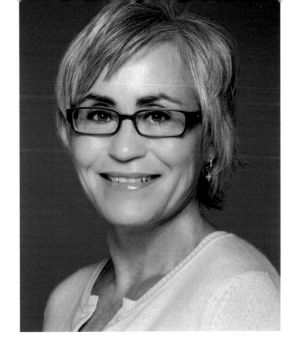

JOEY is one of those lucky women who looks amazing with naturally gray hair. "There's a beauty in embracing what you have naturally and making the most of it," she says. Her only complaint about her hair is that it has a tendency to turn yellow. She already has a violet shampoo, but she's not keeping it in her hair long enough to make a difference. I told her to let the shampoo sit in her hair the entire time she's in the shower—about ten minutes will do the trick.

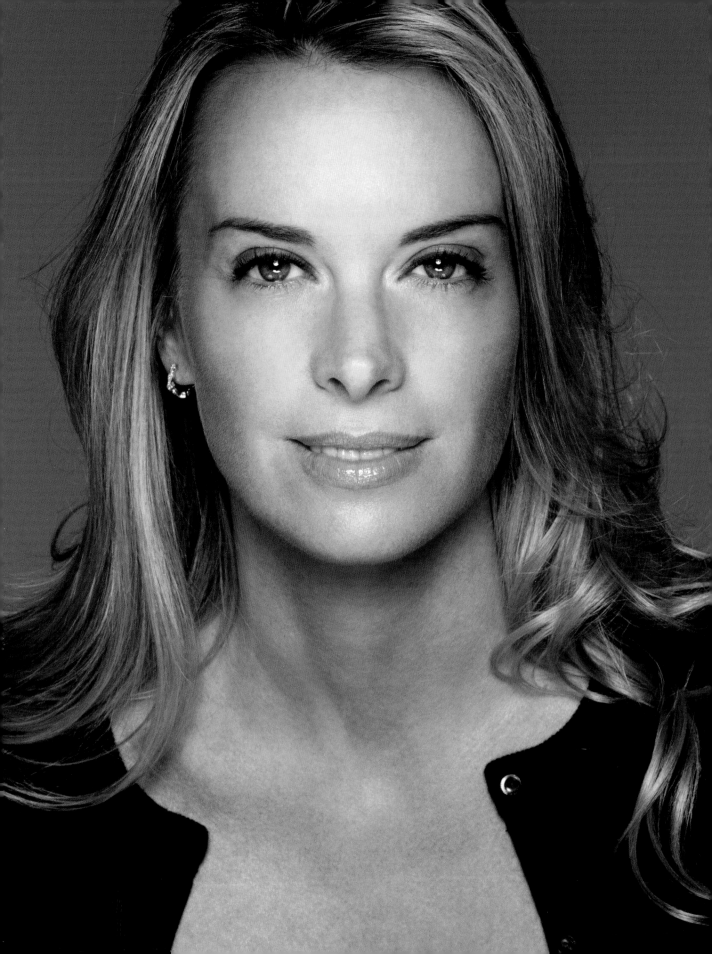

Highlights
The Instant Face Brightener

Mario says that most people are born with natural highlights—they just happen to fade and darken with age. Done right, highlights can have the same lifting and brightening effect on your face as makeup or a good night's rest. And the good news is that highlights flatter nearly everyone.

Rather than going for allover highlights in one color (this looks flat and overdone), Mario suggests a few strategically placed highlights in the same color family. "For the most natural look, I use warm highlights underneath and toward the back of the head, slightly lighter highlights on top, and lightest highlights toward the front of the head," he says. This gradation in highlights mimics the color your hair turns when you're out in the sun. In addition to casting a pretty glow on the skin, highlights give a haircut more texture and soften the edges of the cut.

Resist the urge to get your highlights redone every month—you'll just end up looking overprocessed. Touch-ups every three months are more than enough. If you're thinking of getting highlights, some flattering shade suggestions appear opposite.

HAIR COLOR HIGHLIGHTS

BLONDE
You can go anywhere from three to six shades lighter than your hair color. If you're a dirty blonde, choose cool tones like icy blonde. If you're a golden blonde, you can blend gold and beige highlights.

LIGHT TO MEDIUM BROWN
Golden highlights. To avoid a stripey look, don't go more than two to three shades lighter than your hair color.

BLACK
Warm tones like caramel. Don't go more than two to three shades lighter than your hair color.

REDHEAD
You already have natural highlights, so give your hair dimension with lowlights that are one to two shades darker than your hair color. What's the difference between highlights and lowlights? Highlights brighten your base color and lowlights darken your base color. The best way to avoid obvious roots is with a combination of highlights and lowlights.

Eyebrows
Should They Match Your Hair Color?

If you've made a subtle change in your hair color, simply tweak the shade of powder shadow or brow pencil that you normally use to define your brows. There's a flattering brow color for every hair color; refer to Chapter 3 for shade suggestions.

But if you are changing your hair color dramatically (for example, going from dark brown to light blonde), it's a good idea to dye your brows to match your new "do." If you're coloring your hair at the salon, ask your colorist to do your brows as well. You can dye your brows at home, but be careful not to get any hair dye in your eyes. It takes some trial and error to figure out how long to keep the dye on to achieve a brow color that complements your hair. When in doubt, wash the dye off sooner rather than later (you can always reapply the dye!).

IN BETWEEN APPOINTMENTS?
TRY BOBBI'S QUICK COLOR FIXES

———◆———

I've discovered a few products in my makeup bag that do a decent job of covering gray roots for the day: dense powder eye shadow that matches your hair color (I apply it with a full eye-shadow brush); brown mascara (if you use it in your hair, don't use the same tube on your lashes); and brown gel eyeliner (also applied with the same eye-shadow brush I mentioned earlier).

Try an at-home hair dye that's semipermanent and peroxide-free. I always get good results with a product called Beautiful Collection by Clairol Professional.

When I don't want to dye my entire head, I use root-only color. Nice 'n Easy's Root Touch-up takes just ten minutes and it comes with a mini brush that gets even hard-to-reach hairs.

Check your local beauty supply store for hair crayons or hair color wands. They're easy to apply (simply draw or brush color onto hair using light strokes) and wash out when you shampoo your hair. A good one to try is Color-Mark, which comes in 12 shades to match most permanent hair colors.

———————

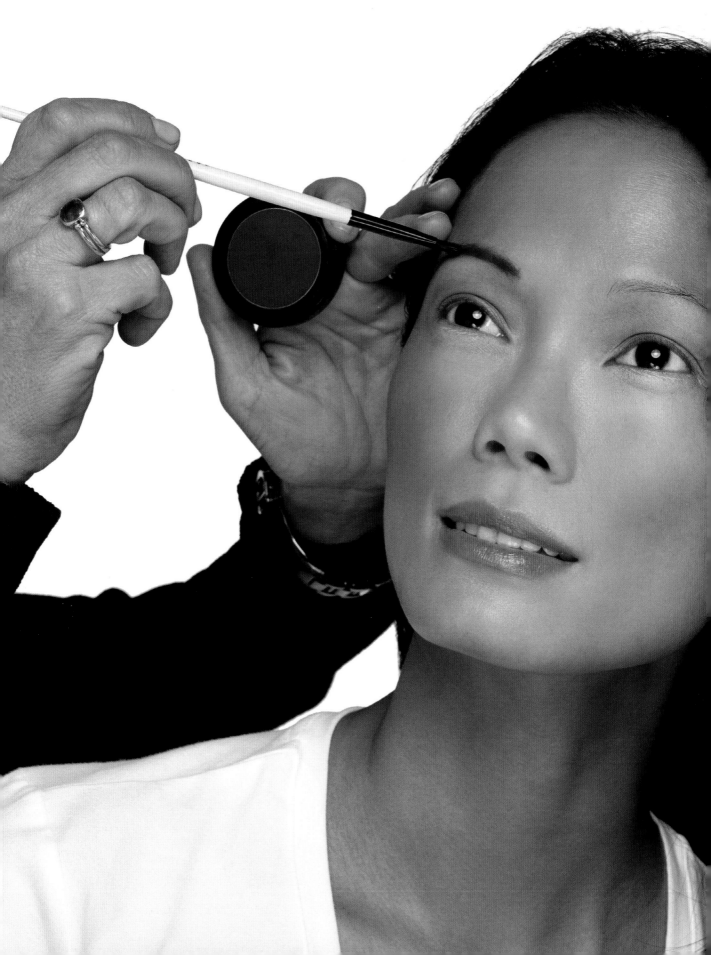

A Makeup Palette for Every Hair Color

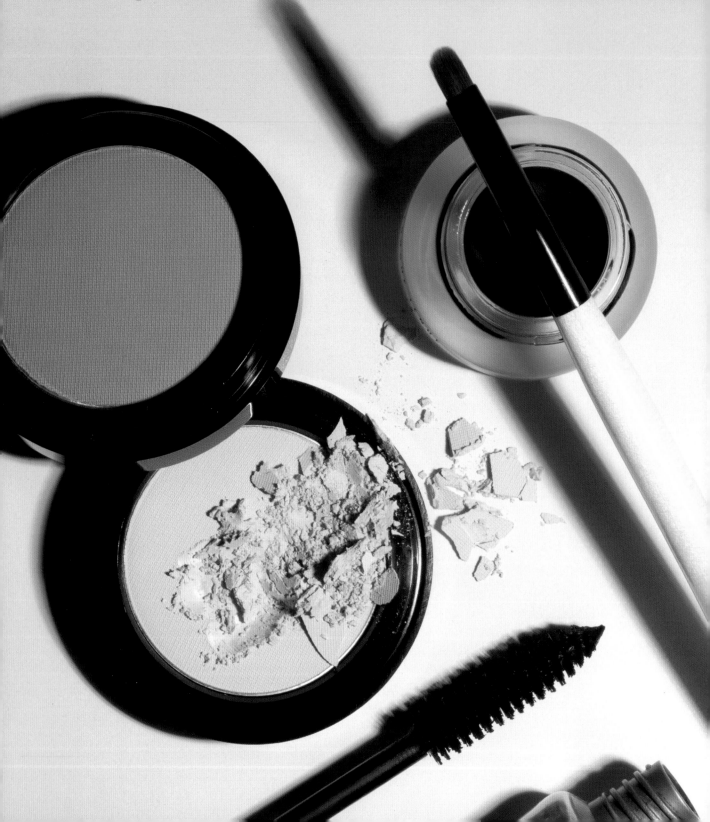

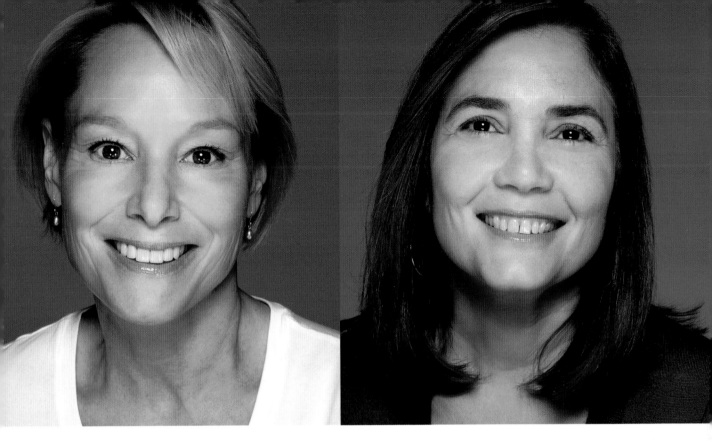

Blonde Hair

Blondes look best in soft, pastel makeup shades that complement the lightness of their hair color. Dark makeup shades are an overly harsh contrast and will make you look too hard.

Eyes Pick bone, ash, or petal eye shadows and dark brown liner.

Cheeks Try pale pink or nectar shades of blush.

Lips Go for light to medium tones of pink, peach, or rose.

Light Brown Hair

Light brown hair has a tendency to give skin a lackluster look, so brighten things up with medium neutrals and sheer brights (natural-looking highlights work great too).

Eyes Pick bone and taupe eye shadows and mahogany liner.

Cheeks Choose pale pink, sand pink, and tawny shades of blush.

Lips Try pinky browns, soft shades of rose, and sheer berries.

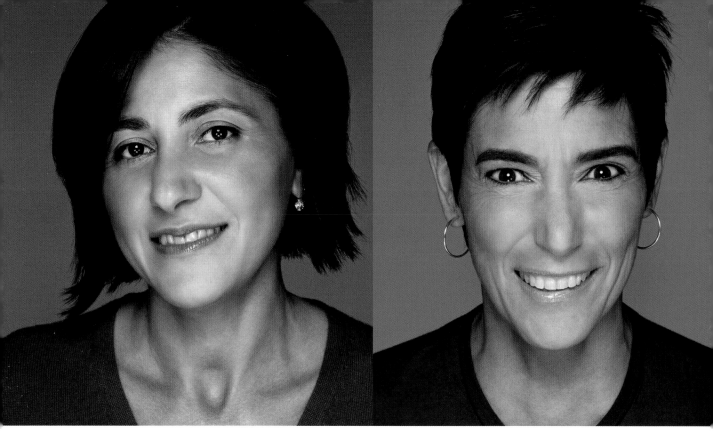

Medium Brown Hair

Medium brown hair tends to give the skin a monochromatic look, so create subtle contrasts with medium neutrals and brights.

Eyes Try bone, beige, and gray eye shadows and medium brown liner.

Cheeks Go for pale pink, flushed pink, and pinky brown shades of blush.

Lips Choose pinky browns, rosy pink, and sheer reds.

Dark Brown to Black Hair

Dark brown and black hair can make skin look pale, so you need to add color to your face to counteract this.

Eyes Pick bone, light brown, or mocha eye shadows and dark brown to charcoal liner.

Cheeks Try rosy pink, brownish pink, or rosy brown shades of blush.

Lips Go for pinky browns, plum browns, or blue reds.

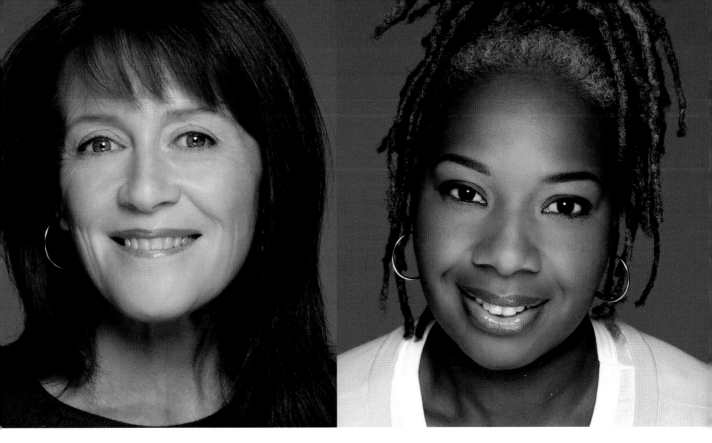

Red Hair

The burnt-amber tone of your hair will warm up your complexion, so your makeup should complement this.

Eyes Pick bone, taupe, or mossy green eye shadows and red brown to dark brown liner.

Cheeks Try medium brown, rosy brown, or apricot shades of blush.

Lips Go for peach, light brown, brownish pink, or red.

White/Gray Hair

Gray hair can drain color from your face, leaving you looking washed out. Brighter makeup colors in cool tones will give your face a lift.

Eyes For blue eyes, pick white and gray eye shadows and slate or navy liner. For brown or green eyes, stick to more neutral shades of eye shadow.

Cheeks Try soft pink or coral shades of blush.

Lips Go for nude, rose, pink, coral, or red—any colors that give the face a lift.

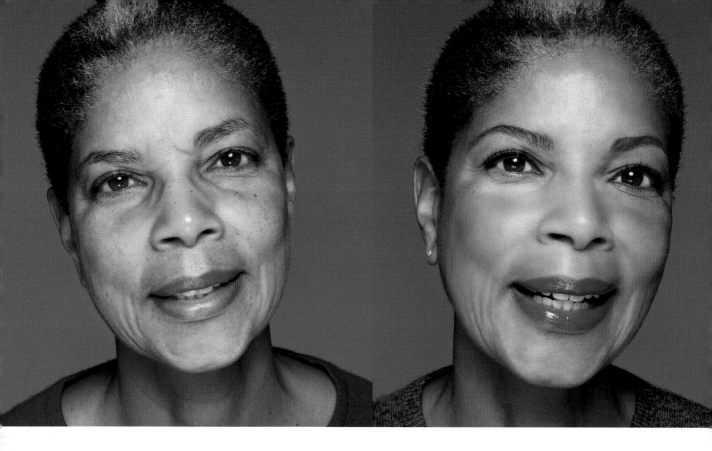

Two Takes on Gorgeous

Though Sharon loved being gray, she wondered what she would look like if she colored her hair. We dyed her hair a dark ash brown and she loved the results. Sharon's new hair color called for an updated makeup palette. She needed richer tones, so we warmed up her face with bronzing powder and a sheer maple brown lip tint. Before she looked gorgeous and distinguished...now she looks just plain gorgeous!

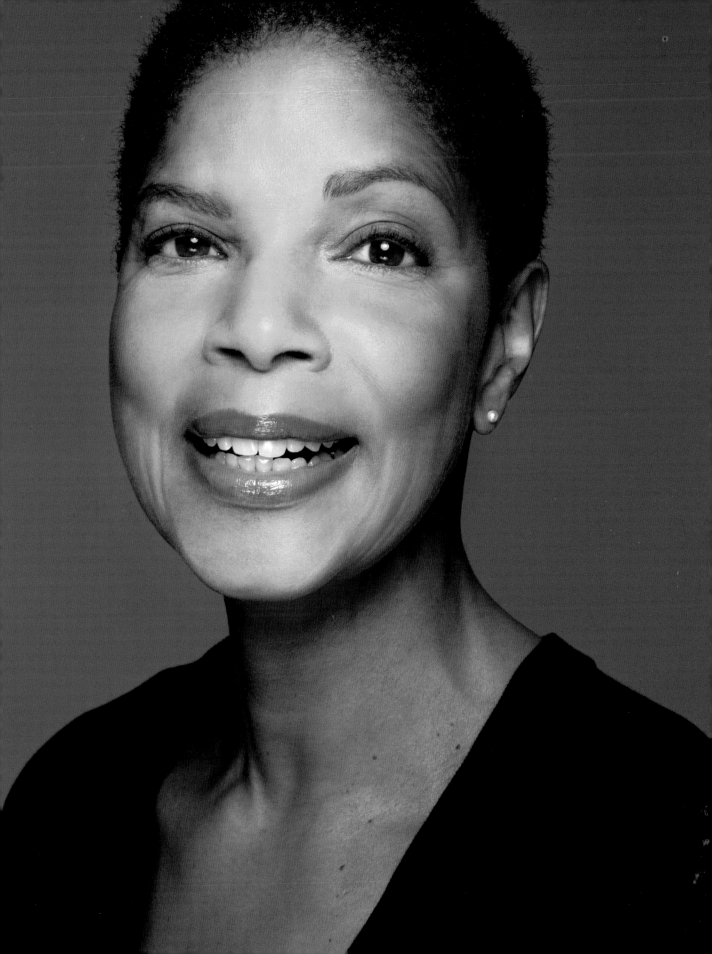

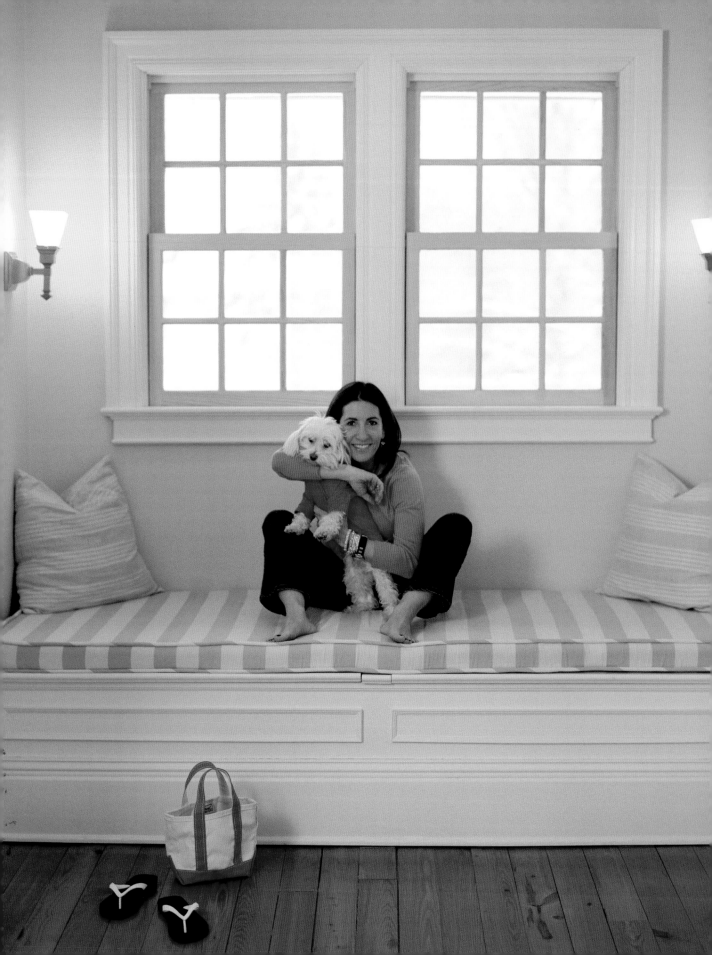

CHAPTER 5

INSTANT UPDATES

Unexpected Ways to Turn Back the Hands of Time

I am forever editing and cleaning out my closets in an effort to wean myself down to a few key pieces. But the truth is that I can never resist buying another navy suit or pair of black pants—after all, this pair of black pants might be "the one" that I've been searching for all along. And when it comes to undergarments, I am continually on the hunt for better bras and panties that are both pretty and flattering.

The reason that I'm so obsessed with getting a perfect wardrobe is that my body changes day to day and week to week. Hormonal fluctuations and water retention can wreak havoc on my body and the way clothes fit me. The suit that buttons comfortably one day suddenly makes me feel like a stuffed sausage two days later. This used to drive me crazy until I decided to stock my closet with a few different sizes of clothes and undergarments. So on days when I'm feeling bigger, instead of squeezing myself into a too-tight pair of pants, I'll wear a bigger size (no one knows except me).

Over the years I've picked up tips like these (and many more!) from the talented stylists and fashion experts I work with every day. In this chapter, I'll share some of my favorite tricks—from finding the perfect bra, to knowing what clothes flatter your figure, to brightening up your face with teeth whitening or a pair of sparkly earrings.

Start with a Good Foundation

A good foundation isn't necessary only for your face. Having been naturally "blessed" with a large chest, I've had a lifelong obsession with finding the right bra. I think smaller breasts make you look thinner, make clothes look better, and make it much easier to exercise (which is why I've never understood why women get breast implants). Over the years, I've discovered the importance of undergarments that smooth, lift, and support. I'm not talking about the dowdy old-school numbers that our grandmothers wore. Today there are actually many options that are both flattering and natural looking.

I have acquired a whole wardrobe of undergarments because I believe that looking good starts with the very first thing you put on. Life isn't a dress rehearsal—I want to wear underwear that makes me feel good every day. I have underwire bras with smooth, rounded cups that minimize for everyday wear, bra extenders for my premenstrual days, and demi-cup bras for special occasions. Visible panty lines are not pretty, so I've stocked up on thongs that fit comfortably and briefs that give me a smooth line. I also have looser briefs for days when I feel bloated.

One of my frequent shopping haunts for undergarments is Johari, a Montclair, New Jersey, boutique owned by Deborah Furr. Deborah believes that undergarments can make or break an outfit. "I can tell when a woman isn't wearing the right bra or underwear because her clothes don't fall properly," says Deborah. "When a woman wears the right undergarments, she looks thinner, her breasts look more lifted, and her clothes look better on her." Here are some of the helpful pointers Deborah has shared with me:

Check your bra measurements every six months to make sure your bra still fits you correctly. Breasts will change in size and shape many times over the course of your life as a result of pregnancy, weight gain, weight loss, and aging. Some women see significant changes going through their monthly cycle.

When shopping for a bra, focus on how it fits you rather than on the size of the cup and the band. You may not be the same size in all bras because cup and band size vary depending on where the bra is manufactured, for example, European bras generally run smaller than American bras.

A bra fits you properly if the band feels snug, but not tight. The band will stretch about half an inch during wear, so allow room to move. Each of the breasts should fill the cup, but not spill out. If you're big-breasted, the bra should lift your breasts off your rib cage. Adjust the straps of the bra each time you wear the bra. Pull the straps as tight as you can without cutting into your skin.

Don't limit yourself to one bra style. Every woman should own at least three styles: a day bra (also known as the "T-shirt bra") that offers support and camouflages nipples, a sports bra to keep breasts from jiggling during workouts, and a plunge or strapless bra for formal attire. When buying a bra, consider what type of clothing you plan on wearing with the bra.

Adjust your bra for the most flattering fit. To avoid the unsightly "back fat" effect (caused when the bra is fastened too tightly) try fastening your bra on the middle hook—this will give you enough support without fitting too snugly. If you still don't have a smooth line, try a seamless bra (companies like Wacoal make laser-cut bras that don't have any seams), a bra with a wider band that has extra support panels, or a tank top with built-in control panels.

If you're wearing a slim-fitting outfit or an unforgiving knit, you can camouflage bulges with a body smoother by companies like BodyWrap and SPANX. Try a tank or T-shirt-style top if you have love handles. A boy-cut short helps control stomach and hip bulges and can be worn under both pants and skirts. Don't be afraid to layer.

A BOBBI POINTER: THE SAFETY-PIN TRICK

———◆———

I've learned many great tricks working with magazine and television stylists over the years. One of my favorites is the "safety-pin trick" because it gives an instantly slimming effect (invaluable for when I make television appearances or get my picture taken). Here's how to do it: pull your bra straps together at the back and safety pin them together. This simple adjustment will lift your chest and make you look like you've dropped about five pounds.

———

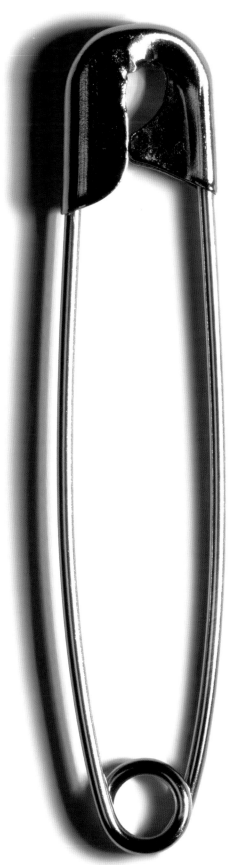

Dress for Your Style—and Your Body

Comfort is my top priority when I dress. I've figured out what works for me and I stick to it. I've never been about avant-garde or funky looks, and I've always felt most at ease in clean, simple styles. Through some trial and error I've learned that I look best in fitted jackets (I drown in loose, tunic-style jackets), pants with narrow legs that flare slightly at the bottom, and slim-cut sweaters. I used to think that I could wear only cropped sweaters (since I'm so petite), but I've recently discovered that slightly longer styles actually make me look taller. I'm drawn to neutral colors like navy, brown, black, white, and gray—but every once in a while I like to add a shot of color like bright pink or French blue.

I've always admired women whose clothes reflect their personal style. As I get older, women who dress young and fresh (but who don't look like they're trying to compete with their daughter's style) inspire me. Whenever I need help with an outfit for a special event, I call my friend and celebrity stylist Deborah Medeiros-Baker. Deborah's got dressing down to a science. She knows how to pick clothes to make any woman look and feel good, so I asked her to share her secrets:

I think that it's important to be comfortable in your clothes—but remember that comfortable doesn't mean sloppy. You can never go wrong if you keep it simple and elegant. This is a time when less is more! Opt for the best fabrics (wear cashmere whenever possible) and shoes that your budget allows. Stay aware of the trends without following them too literally. Evaluate your wardrobe on a regular basis (one to two times a year) and get rid of anything that is worn out and shows signs of aging (unless it's an invaluable vintage piece). If an item of clothing or pair of shoes isn't comfortable or if you haven't worn it in the last two years, it's time to let it go. Organizations like Dress for Success (visit www.dressforsuccess.org for information) will gladly accept gently worn business attire and accessories.

Undergarments are crucial, especially at this age when we start to see sagging and lumps that we didn't have before. The right bra and bodywear will lift and give you a smoother look. Footless stockings (try SPANX) are perfect under jeans, pants, and skirts. Under dresses I suggest one-piece body smoothers with short-style bottoms (I like the ones by Nancy Gantz). Lycra camisoles (Sassybax, SPANX, Only Hearts, and Hanro make the best ones) work wonders and are totally imperceptible under shirts, blouses, and sweaters.

The most flattering fabrics are those with texture and body. Knits, matte jersey, and different gauges of wool are forgiving and they drape well without clinging. Stay away from fabrics like charmeuse, satin, and some silks because they have a tendency to accentuate dimples and bumps. Don't be afraid of prints. You're always safe going with a midsize print (microprints can get too cutesy and bold prints can be overwhelming). Look in the mirror and check your reflection from different angles to make sure that the print flatters you all around. Prints are best worn in moderation, so be sure to balance a printed piece with something solid.

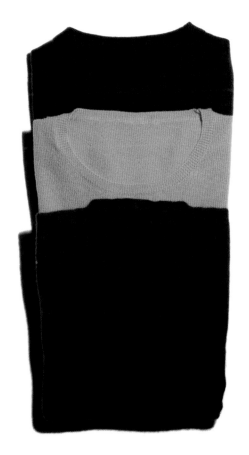

QUICK-FIX KIT

◆

This kit comes in handy when you're on the go and the unexpected—a spill, undone hem, broken bra clasp—happens.

Prewrapped wipes (to disinfect your hands and remove food and makeup stains).

Safety pins in silver and black (great for fixing a dropped hem, a bra or popped button, even the clasp on a necklace).

Wig tape or double-stick tape (to keep your neckline in place and prevent bra straps from showing). You can also use the tape to remove lint and dog hair.

A pair of tiny fold-up scissors and a sewing kit with prethreaded needles.

A small bottle of body lotion for those last-minute situations when you notice your cuticles are ragged or your elbows look ashy.

Bounce sheets, hair spray, or static spray to get rid of static cling on clothes.

A non-oily eye makeup remover will remove most stains. To avoid getting lint on your clothing, use a cotton cloth or makeup sponge to blot on the remover.

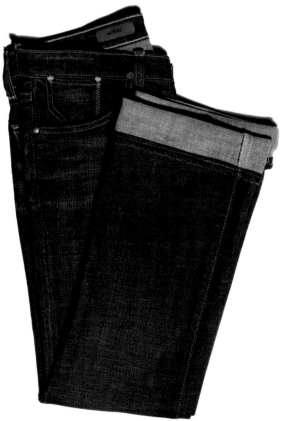

The Perfect Wardrobe: Key Basics to Invest In

Undergarments Seamless bras (black and nude), sexy black lace bra and panty set, sports bras, thongs (black and nude), lace-trimmed camisoles (black, white, and nude), Lycra camisoles (black and nude), one-piece body smoother with long legs (nude and/or black), nude footless pantyhose.

Tops Good-quality cotton Ts (black, white, and a handful of fun colors), cotton ribbed tank tops (black, white, and some colors), black fitted turtleneck, black cardigan, comfy crew-neck or V-neck sweater, two or three crisp white blouses, sexy evening camisole top, simple black dress.

Bottoms Two or more pairs of great-fitting jeans, white denim jeans, slim black well-tailored pants, form-fitting skirt.

Suits One to two well-cut fitted suits in black or navy. You can also wear the jacket and pants as separates.

Jackets and coats Jean jacket, blazers (use them as accessories—try different colors or textures, velvet, leather), wool or cashmere coat, down jacket, trench coat.

Shoes and handbags Black low-heel sling-back pumps, colored high-heel sling-back pumps or sandals, gold or silver metallic high-heel sandals, ballet slippers (black or metallic), comfy flat shoes (driving mocs and loafers), suede or leather tall boots, sneakers (trendy and exercise), flip-flops, waterproof boots (Wellies), a designer handbag (or two).

Jewelry and accessories A great watch, diamond stud earrings (real and/or fake), silver or gold hoop earrings, chandelier earrings, tiny pearl or gem drop earrings, a pair of fabulous sunglasses, a cashmere wrap.

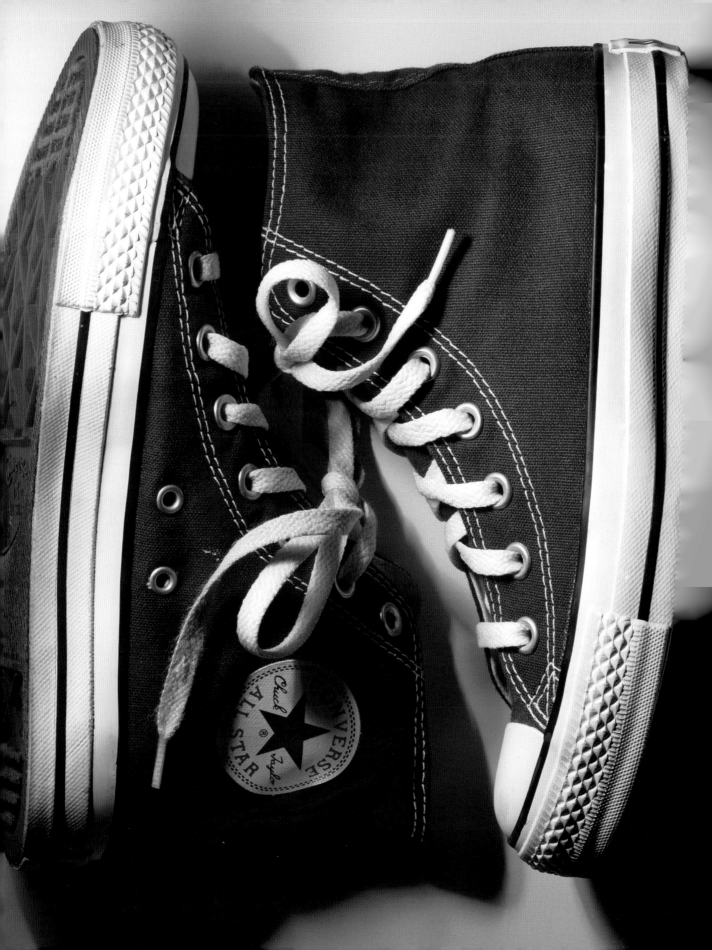

Figure-Fixing Clothes

If you have an ample bottom or fuller hips It's all about fabrics that have stretch! Choose long, slim-cut tops (layer them) that cover part of your bottom. Go for pants with a fitted thigh and slight flare at the bottom, and avoid straight and tapered legs. Opt for A-line skirts and dresses and add a heeled, pointy-toe shoe.

If you have narrow hips Create the illusion of curves with empire-cut tops and dresses, full skirts or tiered skirts, and fitted pants that are flared at the bottom (avoid straight-leg pants—they'll just emphasize your narrow frame).

If you have short legs Avoid capris and go for straight-leg pants that flare at the bottom. Skip ankle-strap shoes in favor of sling-backs and heeled or wedged sandals. Choose shoe colors that blend with the color of your pants to help elongate your legs.

If you're short-waisted Wear skirts, pants, and belts low on your waist to create a longer-looking torso. Avoid anything that cuts your natural waistline. If a top is too short, pair it with a longer tank underneath. An empire top with a fitted bust is a great option because it draws your attention up and away from your waist.

If you have a long torso Choose skirts and pants with wider waistbands and wear them on your waistline (not on your hips). Wrap dressing (sweaters and dresses) is a great way to break up a long torso and bring attention to the waist.

If you have a thick middle Start with undergarments that smooth and hold you in. A fitted blazer or wrap dress is a great way to cinch you and create the illusion of a leaner midsection. If you prefer to draw attention away from your middle, wear dark colors on top and use pretty jewelry to draw attention up toward your face.

If you're large-breasted A minimizing bra will create the illusion of a smaller bust while still enhancing your shape. Wear a smoothing camisole under your clothing to create clean, smooth lines. Choose fitted and tailored blouses, jackets, and dresses over large, unstructured tops. Stick to solid and darker color tops. Ballet necklines are very flattering because they emphasize your décolletage while covering the bust line. Layering with a cardigan or jacket is another way to visually minimize a fuller bust.

Get It Tailored to Fit

Although I am only five feet tall, I am by no means a waif. I am more muscular than lithe, and my chest is ample. As a result, clothes that I buy off the rack seldom fit me properly. Since custom tailoring is prohibitively expensive, I bring my off-the-rack purchases to my neighborhood tailor, Anna Chiommino, for minor alterations. Anna takes the shoulders in on my jackets and hems my pants so that they don't drag, but are still long enough to create the illusion of height. In addition to making minor tweaks, a good tailor can also modernize out-of-date pieces (like your circa 1980s blazer) that you just can't bear to part with. Anna shares her expert tailoring tips below:

A fitted blazer is an easy way to accentuate your waistline. When you get a jacket taken in, be sure to button it before the tailor pins it. This will ensure that he or she doesn't take too much in. You should be able to fasten the middle button (the button that hits your waistline) without any tugging.

The waistband on your pants and skirts should never be so tight that you spill over it. There should be enough allowance for you to be able to slip your thumb into the waistband easily.

When it comes to skirt hemlines, you can never go wrong with a hem that hovers around the knee (this can be just above the knee, mid-knee, or just below the knee). This is a classic length that flatters all body types. After a certain age you shouldn't wear skirts that are too short.

Avoid pleats at all costs. They do not, as some women think, camouflage a big stomach. Pleats actually do the opposite and tend to create a ballooning effect. If you're concerned about your midsection, choose flat-front pants without darts.

If you're petite, stay away from cuffed pants because they cut you off and make you look shorter. Cuffless pants will give you a longer look and create the illusion of height.

Straight-leg pants with a slight flare at the bottom flatter all body types. A tapered leg is OK on someone with a slim, small build—but it totally works against a woman who is bottom-heavy.

A BOBBI POINTER: TAILORING TIP

I've been taking my bras to the tailor for years. Because I have a small frame and a large chest, most bra straps are too long and fall off my shoulders. I ask the tailor to shorten the straps by about an inch and the bra fits me perfectly.

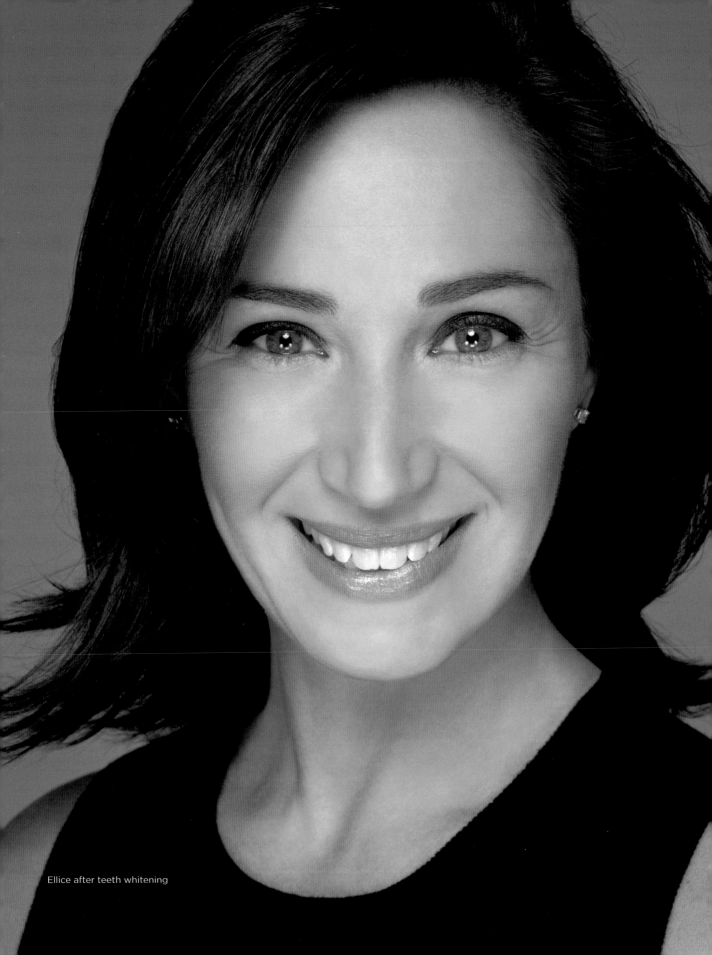

Ellice after teeth whitening

Give Yourself Something to Smile About

After my second book came out I decided to treat myself to teeth whitening at BriteSmile. The procedure, which uses gel and light instead of heat or lasers, was pretty new to the market, so it was definitely a bit of a splurge at the time. But it was well worth it. Looking in the mirror afterward, I was pleasantly surprised to see that getting my teeth whitened not only brought out the whites in my eyes, but it also made my entire face look younger and brighter. I was hooked.

Over the years I tried other teeth-whitening methods and got varying results. My dentist made me a custom-fitted mouth guard designed to be worn a few hours a day. The upside was that it cost about half as much as the BriteSmile procedure. The downside was that I didn't see the results immediately. I also tried over-the-counter mouth guards and coated strips and found that they didn't dramatically change the color of my teeth. At best, they were a good way to maintain my teeth after a whitening session. I've gotten the most noticeable results with professional teeth whitening and I think that it's worth saving up for.

Here's what you can expect if you're thinking about the procedure: the dentist starts by applying a hydrogen peroxide–based bleaching gel to your teeth. Next, the gel is "activated" by a special blue light. The gel is reapplied every twenty minutes for a total of one hour—and you're done. Your teeth may feel a little sensitive for the first twenty-four hours, so avoid very hot or cold drinks and take some aspirin. Since your teeth are more porous after the treatment, you should also avoid red wine and coffee (both will restain your teeth) during this initial twenty-four-hour period.

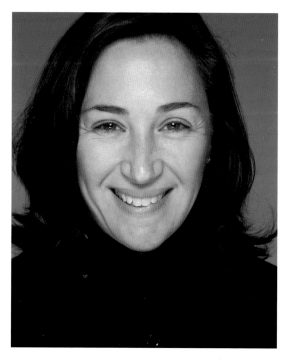

Ellice before teeth whitening

A BOBBI POINTER: SMILE SAVER

Walking through my offices in the morning, I often spot coworkers sipping their hot coffee through straws. After weeks of wondering, I finally asked one of the women about the straw. She replied that the straw keeps her teeth from getting stained by the caffeine in the coffee. Other tooth stainers include tea, red wine, and smoking (which we all know is both a beauty and health no-no).

Jewelry as Makeup

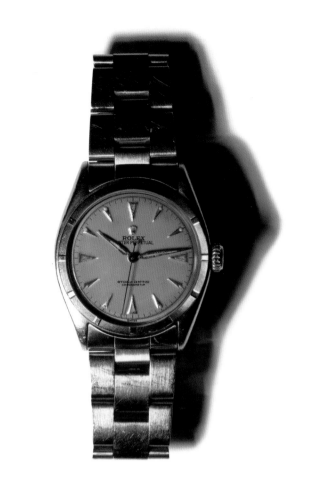

A few years ago I received a pair of pink pearl earrings for my birthday. I instantly fell in love with these earrings because of the way the pink tones of the pearls magically brought out the natural pink in my cheeks. Now, whenever I feel under the weather or need a lift, I reach for my pearls.

The next time you put on a pair of earrings, pay attention to the way the color of the earrings affects your face. Pearls and diamonds (they're a girl's best friend for a reason) cast a flattering glow on all complexions. And I love how colored gemstones can enhance the color of any woman's eyes. Clear emerald and light emerald earrings make green and hazel eyes pop. If you have blue eyes, you can make them stand out even more with pale turquoise or ocean blue gemstones. Choose amber and topaz gemstones or southwestern turquoise if you have brown eyes. Have fun with your jewelry—any great colored jewelry will add to your beauty. Plus, it's prettier and more modern to wear pale blue earrings than pale blue eye shadow!

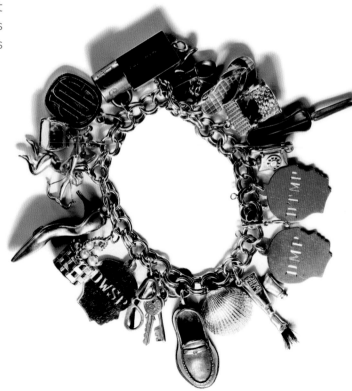

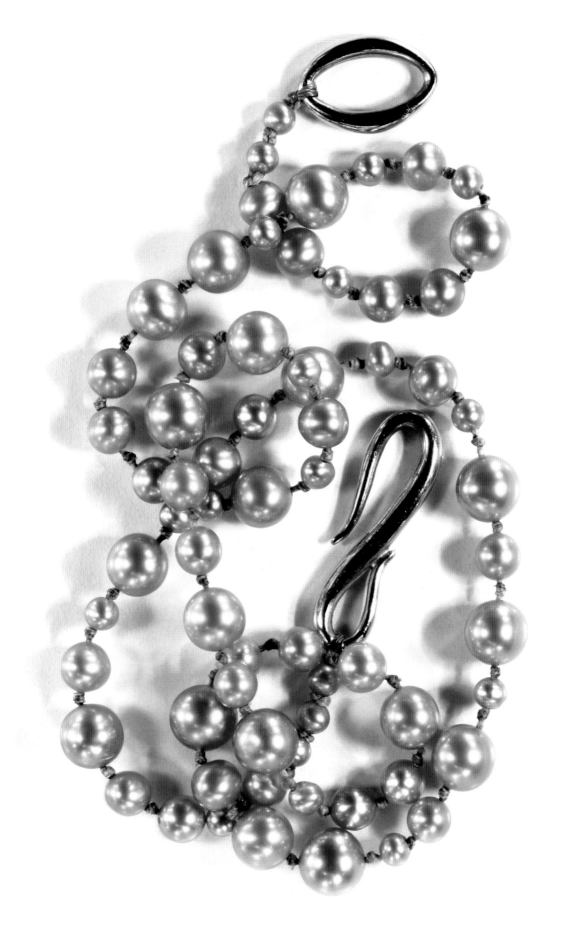

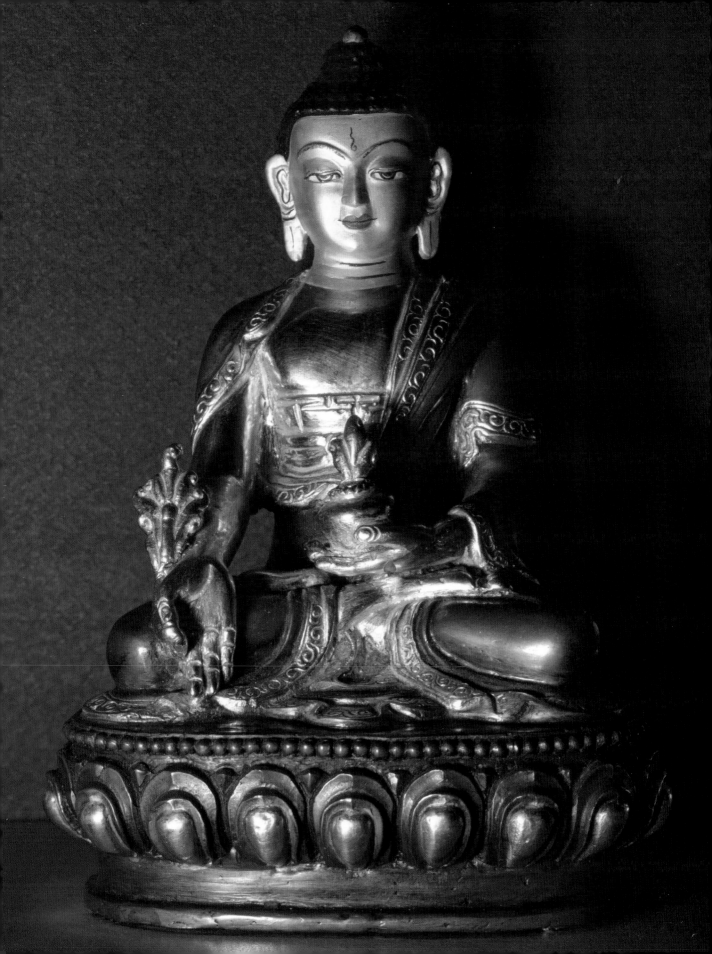

CHAPTER 6

MENOPAUSE
Dealing with "The Change"—Beautifully

When I got my period at the age of eleven, I had no idea that I was beginning a lifelong descent into hormone hell. As a teenager and young adult, I dealt with bloating, mood swings, and occasional pimples for a good week out of every month. Then came the baby-making years of my thirties. I gave birth to my last child when I was forty-one—and I was still in full child-rearing mode when my body started its next transition.

For me, the change came on slowly. At first I just didn't feel good and I was tired all the time. I started crying while watching commercials and I wasn't in the mood to talk to even my best friends. I also started to notice changes in my appearance. My skin felt dry, no matter what I put on my face. The jeans that had always fit me perfectly were inexplicably tight (even though I hadn't changed my diet or exercise routine). I was at a complete loss as to how to deal with what was happening to me.

This all changed when I picked up *The Wisdom of Menopause*, a book by Dr. Christiane Northrup. It was full of information on the changes that I was experiencing and what my choices were for dealing with the different physical and emotional issues. I started eating beauty foods like edamame (soybeans) and walnuts, and I went to a nutritionist to learn what supplements I needed to take. I added face oil to my beauty routine (I layered it with my regular face moisturizer for intense hydration). And finally, I went on an individualized form of hormone replacement therapy called bioidentical hormone replacement therapy (BHRT).

The best advice that I got from Dr. Northrup's book is that perception is everything. Menopause can be a positive experience if you choose to be positive about it. This is a time when you have to listen to your body, not just to your head. Slow down and be kind to yourself. And most important, pay attention and be open to the changes that come your way.

A New Perspective on Menopause

Often referred to as "the change of life" or "the change," menopause occurs when your ovaries produce so little estrogen that you no longer get your period. Technically speaking, you're in menopause when you haven't gotten your period for twelve straight months (in the United States, the average age for women hitting menopause is fifty-one). The journey to menopause starts with perimenopause, when estrogen production slowly decreases. You'll start to experience symptoms like irregular periods, hot flashes, and mood swings. According to my gynecologist Dr. Gerald Ciciola, one of the most common misconceptions that women have about menopause is that it's a sudden stop rather than a gradual process. "There isn't an instant cookie-cutter answer to dealing with menopause. It takes time to individualize how you're feeling and how it will affect your day-to-day life," says Dr. Ciciola. "The next misconception is that menopause is some sort of disease rather than a natural and positive process of life. Menopause should be seen as a time for calmness."

Five Natural Ways to Deal with the Change

1. Breathe. Consider taking up yoga.
2. Add soy-based foods to your diet and improve your overall diet.
3. Dress in layers and wear cotton clothes.
4. Exercise regularly.
5. Sleep in a cool, well-ventilated room.

Wise Words from Christiane Northrup, M.D.

"Menopause can be the beginning of the very best years of a woman's life if she is willing to update her beliefs about what is possible. The hormonal shifts that characterize perimenopause are invariably accompanied by emotional and mental shifts that are designed to bring up old unfinished business from our pasts, which we need to process and discard once and for all. Chief among those outmoded beliefs is the notion that midlife women are no longer sexy, desirable, and beautiful. Nothing could be further from the truth! During midlife, we all come to an uncompromising crossroads. One path says 'grow.' The other says 'die.' When we cling to old, outmoded habits, beliefs, and behaviors that no longer serve us, the risk of chronic disease increases dramatically. On the other hand, when we have the courage to live authentically from the inside out—heeding our inner wisdom and the dictates of our souls—we have the opportunity to revitalize every cell in our bodies and every aspect of our lives.

"Our souls speak to us insistently during perimenopause through our passions and desires. That is why so many midlife women start new careers, leave dead-end relationships, remodel their homes, move, or in some other way reinvent themselves. Living passionate and pleasurable lives enhances our physical health. That's why those who are deeply in touch with their soul's passion and purpose have an unmistakable glow.

"My advice to midlife women everywhere is this: Trust your desires and trust your hearts. Understand that you cannot care for anyone else optimally if you are not caring for yourself too. Resolve to care for yourself as well as you would a beloved child. This may or may not include bioidentical hormones. But everyone needs regular exercise, a good supplementation program, and good skin care. Be flexible. You can't get it wrong. Your regimen will require updating periodically as you grow and change. Your body, mind, and spirit are going through rebirth—which inevitably will include some labor pains. Be a good midwife to yourself. Be patient. You have years and years ahead of you. This is just the beginning."

Individualizing Hormone Replacement Therapy

In 2002 we were bombarded by media coverage of the Women's Health Initiative Trial. The stories called out the great risks of traditional hormone replacement therapy (HRT), including an increased risk for breast cancer, heart disease, and stroke. Many women I knew were so scared by the reports that they immediately went off HRT—and their harsh menopause symptoms returned. Other women chose to stay on HRT, deciding that quality of life trumped the possible risks. Other women switched to a natural approach that included making better (and healthier) lifestyle choices. The results of the Women's Health Initiative Trial were hotly debated, but one thing became clear: the one-size-fits-all approach of traditional HRT was not only antiquated, but also unhealthy. I, along with many of my girlfriends, struggled to sort through the alternatives.

Then Suzanne Somers came out with a book, *The Sexy Years: Discover the Hormone Connection*, which talked about the individualized form of HRT, bioidentical hormone replacement therapy (BHRT). It sounded too good to be true, but my friends and I were intrigued, so we went online looking for doctors who specialized in this therapy. Our search led us to Dr. Joseph Raffaele of the PhysioAge Medical Group in New York City. From Dr. Raffaele, we learned that BHRT basically adds back the hormones your body has lost. In doing so, BHRT helps the body ward off the symptoms of menopause, including hot flashes, poor sleep, and mood swings, and also helps prevent bone loss.

A Close Look at BHRT

Put simply, bioidentical hormone replacement therapy restores a woman's hormone levels back to youthful levels. BHRT differs from conventional hormone replacement therapy in two very important ways. First, bioidentical hormones are derived from plant sources like yams and soy, and are synthesized to have the same molecular structure as hormones found in the body, such as estradiol, estrone, and estriol. In contrast, conventional hormone replacement therapy uses chemicals that act like hormones, but are not found naturally in the human body (the most commonly used hormones are extracted from the urine of a pregnant mare or are synthetically derived). And second, bioidentical hormones are made by compounding pharmacies on an individualized basis following a prescription from the patient's doctor—in other words, the prescription is customized for each woman. "Every woman experiences menopause differently and has different expectations of what the next thirty or so years will bring in terms of her mental and physical health," says Dr. Raffaele. "Bioidentical hormone replacement therapy gives a woman's body back exactly what it needs—nothing less and nothing more." Side effects, according to Dr. Raffaele, are "virtually eliminated by breaking from traditional HRT and taking only youthful levels of bioidentical estradiol and progesterone, by administering them transdermally, and by monitoring blood levels closely."

BHRT is administered in the form of a cream that you rub into your skin daily (once or twice a day depending on your doctor's instructions). The cream contains three bioidentical hormones—estradiol, progesterone (to offset the risk of uterine cancer from taking estrogen), and testosterone (as a woman ages she also experiences a decline in testosterone, which affects her libido and sense of well-being, and can also lead to weight gain). Doctors prefer the cream form for two reasons: it delivers the hormones directly to the bloodstream (medications that are taken orally go through the liver and change slightly in structure before entering the bloodstream), and it provides steady hormone levels throughout the day, which duplicates the way our ovaries release estrogen. After about six weeks of treatment, your doctor will do a follow-up to check your hormone levels and, if needed, adjust your dosages. Since your body's needs may change over time, you should check in with your doctor after about three months, and then every six months after that.

My friends and I began taking our prescribed doses of BHRT and almost instantly saw and felt improvements. BHRT is not currently considered a mainstream treatment (it's not readily available and it's not covered by insurance), but I strongly believe that the majority of doctors will offer this therapy in the future. Dr. Raffaele agrees: "There's a progression of knowledge about how hormones affect aging and women. In ten to fifteen years almost all women will be on some targeted and tailored form of HRT because it works." If you are considering hormone replacement therapy, do your research. Talk to your gynecologist about your options and read as much as you can. This is truly a time when knowledge is power.

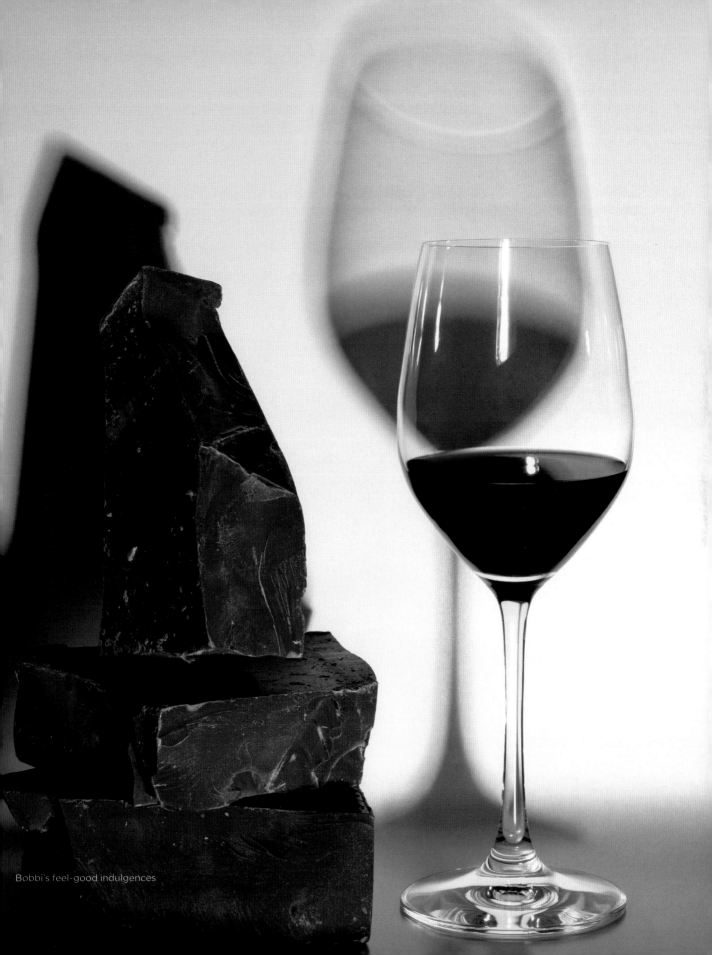

Bobbi's feel-good indulgences

BHRT Case Study
Susan Saunders

I'm forty-six years old, but I've always looked much younger than my age (in fact, people often think that I'm in my thirties). I've always cared about how I look—I was a professional model for twenty-five years and retired a few years ago—and have consistently worked out and maintained a healthy diet.

Perimenopause crept up on me. When I skipped a few periods, the first thing I did was to run out and get a pregnancy test. My skin got very dry, I was tired all the time because I wasn't sleeping, and I put on about five pounds without changing anything. I lost a lot of my self-confidence and I felt like I was PMS-ing all the time.

I mentioned what I was going through to the owner of the gym where I work out, and he said my problems sounded hormone-related. He told me about bioidentical hormones and Dr. Raffaele's practice, so I went online to look for Dr. Raffaele. I also read the book by Suzanne Somers and thought, "That's me."

I didn't know what to expect when I first met with Dr. Raffaele. Women had gotten so scared of hormone replacement therapy and the risk of cancer. But the more I researched, the more I realized that the verdict is overwhelming in support of taking bioidentical hormones.

When I went on BHRT I felt like myself again. I lost 2 percent body fat and went back to my original weight. My skin stopped feeling so dry and dehydrated. I started sleeping like a normal person. My best advice is to do your research and make your own judgment calls. It's unfortunate that we live in a day and age where menopause is still hush-hush. All women go through it, and it seems unfair that we don't talk about it more freely. How you choose to deal with menopause is a very personal choice.

BHRT Case Study
Gayle Friscia

I'm forty-eight now and had a partial hysterectomy (they took out my uterus and left my ovaries) about five years ago. The doctors warned me that there was a slight chance my ovaries would stop functioning. Somewhere around forty-six or forty-seven I started to experience some symptoms of menopause. First I got hot flashes, then I couldn't sleep. Next I got very irritable and felt depressed. This went on for several months, but I put up with it because I came from a family that taught me to deal with pain and discomfort. (When I gave birth to my children, I opted for natural childbirth even though I had the option of an epidural.) I think my turning point came when it got to my head. I felt fuzzy at work and often forgot things. When menopause started to affect my memory and my job, I finally sought help.

When I met with Dr. Raffaele, we talked about everything—what I ate, what supplements I was taking, and what my exercise routine was. In order to find balance, we needed to take everything into consideration. I eat healthy foods (lots of fruits and vegetables and lean meats) and stay away from white foods (pasta and bread). I try to limit my alcohol intake, but occasionally I have red wine or indulge in a bowl of ice cream. I exercise regularly and do a combination of cardio and strength training. BHRT helped me right away. I felt better and looked healthier. I noticed a more even appearance in my skin tone, my wrinkles seemed less pronounced, and my sunspots weren't as dark.

I think the most important thing for women to know is that they don't have to deal with menopause on their own. Don't accept everything your doctor says. When I asked my gynecologist about it, he raised his eyebrows. There's still a lot of skepticism among the mainstream medical community regarding BHRT, so be your own health advocate and trust your instincts.

Beyond BHRT
More Ways to Deal with the Symptoms of Menopause

Problem: A drawn, gaunt-looking face. Also known as face drain, this is the result of lower levels of estrogen that come with age. You'll experience a decline in elastin (which gives skin its elasticity) and collagen (which gives skin its firmness).

Rx: Add life back to skin and give it a plumped-up look with the right mix of skincare products. This is definitely an instance where more is better. Switch from lightweight lotions to richer, more emollient creams and balms. If your face still feels drawn after applying face cream, layer it with a face oil (don't worry, the oil won't clog your pores!).

Problem: Dry skin. This is another side effect of reduced estrogen levels.

Rx: The trick is to add moisture back with face cream or face oil. Look for formulas with hyaluronic acid, which attracts and holds water in the skin. If you have oily skin, use an oil-free moisturizer that will hydrate skin without clogging pores. If you wear makeup, opt for cream-based formulas and skip face powder. After applying makeup, give skin an added glow by gently patting balm on your cheeks.

Problem: Adult acne. This occurs primarily along the chin and neck and is the result of a change in the balance between androgen and estrogen.

Rx: Cleanse skin gently with a nonirritating face wash. Use an exfoliant to get rid of dead skin cells and help encourage skin cell turnover. Treat the blemishes with a topical retinoid like Retin-A. To cover blemishes, use a stick or cream foundation that matches your skin exactly. Spot-apply the cover-up directly on the blemish using a concealer brush or any makeup brush with a small brush head and short, slightly rigid bristles. Gently pat the cover-up with your fingertips to blend it in, then lock it in place with a dusting of sheer face powder.

Problem: Random coarse hairs on the chin. This happens when androgen levels are higher than estrogen levels.

Rx: Tweezing is the fastest way to get rid of individual hairs (I keep tweezers everywhere—my makeup case, car, bathroom, and at work). If you find that you have a particularly noticeable "mustache," you might want to consider waxing. Drugstores sell at-home kits that come with premade strips of wax or meltable wax that's applied with a spatula and then ripped off. If you're leery of the do-it-yourself approach, you can always get waxed by a professional at a spa (you can also check your local nail salons—many now offer waxing services). Try sugaring if you're allergic to waxing. It uses sugar that has a consistency similar to caramel and works the same way as waxing by pulling the hair out from below the surface of the skin. If you want to remove hairs permanently, try electrolysis, which works by killing the hair follicle.

Problem: Thinning hair. This is another side effect of the androgen-to-estrogen ratio leaning in favor of androgen.

Rx: Fill in bare spots with a dark shade of powder eye shadow that's a similar tone to your hair color; use an eye-shadow brush to apply the shadow. To create the illusion of fullness, talk to your hairdresser about getting a haircut with allover layers and short textured pieces (see Chapter 4 for more tips on adding volume). Though it won't grow your hair back 100 percent, you can also try a hair-growth product like Rogaine, which contains minoxidil.

Problem: Dry, lusterless hair. Another side effect of menopause-related hormonal changes.

Rx: Try not to shampoo your hair every day and use a deep conditioner at least twice a week. To get the most benefit out of your conditioner, comb it through your hair when you first get in the shower and leave it in while you soap up and shave. Rinse out the conditioner just before you get out of the shower (the goal is to condition your hair between 10 and 15 minutes). Ask your hairstylist for a hair-gloss treatment to give dull hair a shine boost.

Problem: Hot flashes. When blood vessels expand rapidly, this causes a sudden rise in skin temperature.

Rx: It's all about lifestyle changes. Exercise will help your circulation and your body's ability to adjust to extreme temperature changes. Avoid foods that are known to trigger hot flashes—for example, salty and spicy dishes, hot drinks, alcohol, and caffeinated drinks. Eat products like soybeans, chickpeas, tofu, and soy milk (they contain isoflavones, a plant estrogen similar in structure to the estrogen found in our bodies). Dress in layers so you can easily take off some clothes when a hot flash comes on.

Problem: Poor sleep. A combination of insomnia and waking up in the middle of the night from night sweats can really take a toll on how you feel in the morning.

Rx: Try herbal remedies like passionflower and valerian; taken during the day they can help calm nighttime restlessness and anxiety. Eat dinner before 7:00 p.m. and avoid caffeinated drinks. Instead, try a glass of warm milk or herbal tea. Don't look at the clock when you're in bed or if you wake up in the middle of the night—seeing the numbers tick by will just frustrate you. Try a relaxation technique such as deep abdominal breathing.

Problem: Fuzzy thinking, poor memory, and mood swings. For many women these are the menopause symptoms hardest to deal with.

Rx: Find someone to talk to. Whether it's a girlfriend or a therapist, it's important to have a sounding board. Exercise to clear your mind and release mood-lifting endorphins. Add salmon (it contains omega-3 fatty acids, which are thought to help improve memory) and soy products (soy is thought to boost a neurotransmitter that helps maintain memory) to your diet. Supplements like Saint-John's-wort and ginkgo biloba may also help even out your moods.

OSTEOPOROSIS: PROTECT YOUR BONES

◆

Declining estrogen levels speed up the rate at which your bones lose calcium—which increases your risk for osteoporosis. Here's what you can do to protect yourself.

Bioidentical hormone replacement therapy

Take a calcium supplement: 500 mg in the morning, 500 mg at night taken with 600 mg magnesium.

Eat foods rich in calcium like low-fat yogurt, cheese and milk, tofu, and broccoli.

Drink alcoholic beverages in moderation. Too much alcohol damages the cells that produce new bone and hinders the absorption of vitamin D.

Add weight-bearing exercises to your fitness routine. Turn to Chapter 7 for tips.

———

A Guide to Nutritional Supplements

Dr. Jairo Rodriguez, a nutritionist in New York City, has taught me a lot about the importance of nutritional supplements and how they can help during menopause and beyond. He recommends supplements as part of a healthy, well-balanced diet. If you're new to supplements, start with a multivitamin and add individual vitamins as needed. Dr. Rodriguez says that it's a good idea to begin with the lowest recommended dose (you can always increase the concentration if needed).

Vitamin A Needed for healthy skin. Helps prevent night blindness. Dosage: 10,000 IU daily.

Vitamin B$_6$ Critical in the maintenance of muscle. Dosage: 2.5 mg daily.

Vitamin B$_{12}$ Helps maintain the growth of red blood cells. Dosage: 1,000 mcg daily.

Vitamin C Maintains skin, connective tissue, and elastin (a protein of connective tissue). Dosage: 500 mg daily.

Vitamin E This antioxidant acts to reduce or minimize the trend to atherosclerosis. Dosage: 400 IU daily.

Vitamin D Vital for the functioning of the nervous system. Helps bone growth and maintenance of bone mass during menopause. Dosage: 400 IU daily.

Biotin A deficiency in biotin can result in changes in the skin, as well as hair and weight loss. Dosage: 300 mcg daily, best taken in two doses during the day.

Calcium Reduces risk of osteoporosis, colon cancer, and hypertension. Dosage: 1,200–1,500 mg daily.

Folic acid Folate deficiency can cause anemia. Dosage: 800 mcg daily.

Iron Needed by the body to produce red blood cells and maintain health. Dosage: 10–5 mg daily.

Magnesium Improves calcium absorption. Dosage: 600 mg daily at bedtime.

Niacin Helps improve blood cholesterol levels. Dosage: 50 mg daily.

Pantothenic acid Deficiency can lead to low appetite, skin lesions, and problems metabolizing sugar. Dosage: 100 mg daily.

Riboflavin Necessary for normal cell function, growth, and energy metabolization. Dosage: 50 mg daily.

Selenium Needed for enzymes involved in normal body functions. Dosage: 200 mcg daily.

Thiamin Involved in the nervous system and muscle functions, and necessary for proper digestion. Dosage: 100 mg daily.

Zinc Helps regulate digestion, blood pressure, insulin, and the immune system. Dosage: 50 mg daily.

Midlife Pregnancy
What to Expect When You're Expecting

While some women are experiencing menopause, others are having babies. It's not uncommon today for a woman to have a baby in her forties—I had my youngest son when I was forty-one. There are so many positives about older motherhood—you're old enough to appreciate and enjoy the process, and you're more likely at a point in your life where you have the time and resources to take better care of yourself (like buying nicer pregnancy clothes or treating yourself to a spa weekend!). Dr. Ciciola, my gynecologist, says that a forty-something woman can expect to have a positive experience and a healthy baby if she takes good care of herself going into and during her pregnancy. "While age is a consideration, a woman shouldn't feel like there's a certain age at which she needs to get pregnant. A woman should have a baby at the time in her life that's right for her," he says. "When a woman gets pregnant in her forties, I give her the same basic advice that I give younger women: eat healthy, take your vitamins (especially folic acid, a B vitamin), exercise regularly, limit your caffeine, limit or stop drinking alcohol, and if you're a smoker, stop smoking. Good prenatal care is key."

My sister Linda Arrandt just had her third child at forty-two, so I asked her to share her experience. "I had twins when I was thirty-four. This pregnancy was easier and harder in some ways. It was easier because I wasn't quite as big, but it was harder because I'm eight years older and it took more of a toll on my body. Having been pregnant before, I have more experience to draw from now. I'm less freaked out about things and more easygoing.

"And most of all, I know the importance of having a good support system. When I was younger I was always the first one to offer help, but I had a hard time asking for help myself. I learned how to ask for help when I had the twins, and that lesson stayed with me. If you don't have family around, turn to your friends. It's important to create a support system with the right people.

"I also know how important it is to take care of myself, so I'm eating healthy, taking vitamins and fish oil, and staying away from junky foods, white flour, and too much sugar. And rather than push myself, I listen to what my body needs. So some days my body might say it needs more sleep and other days it might say it needs exercise."

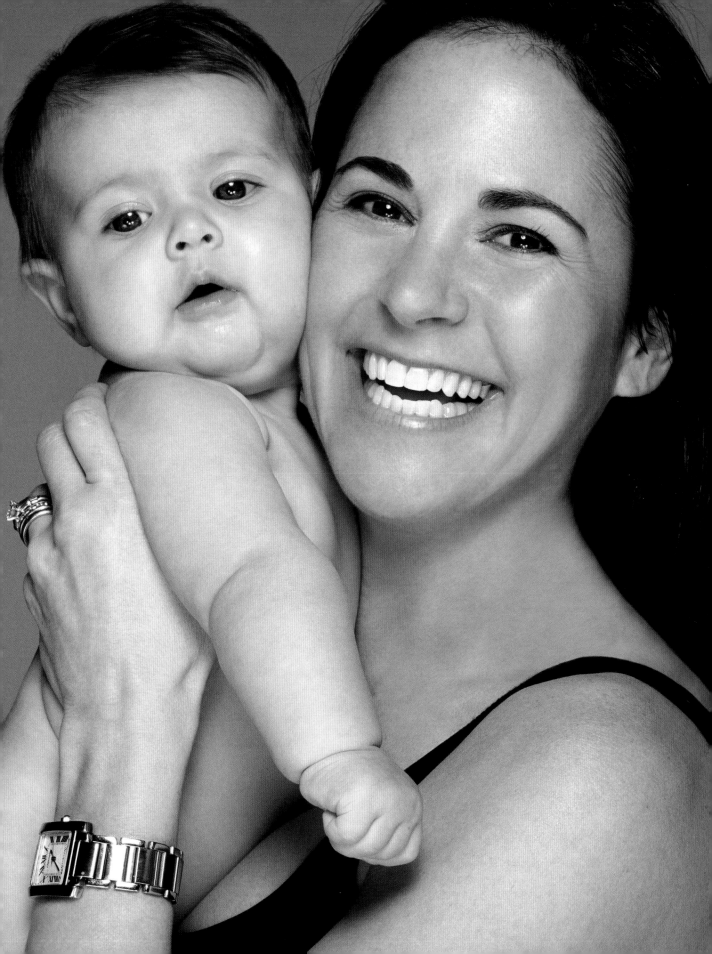

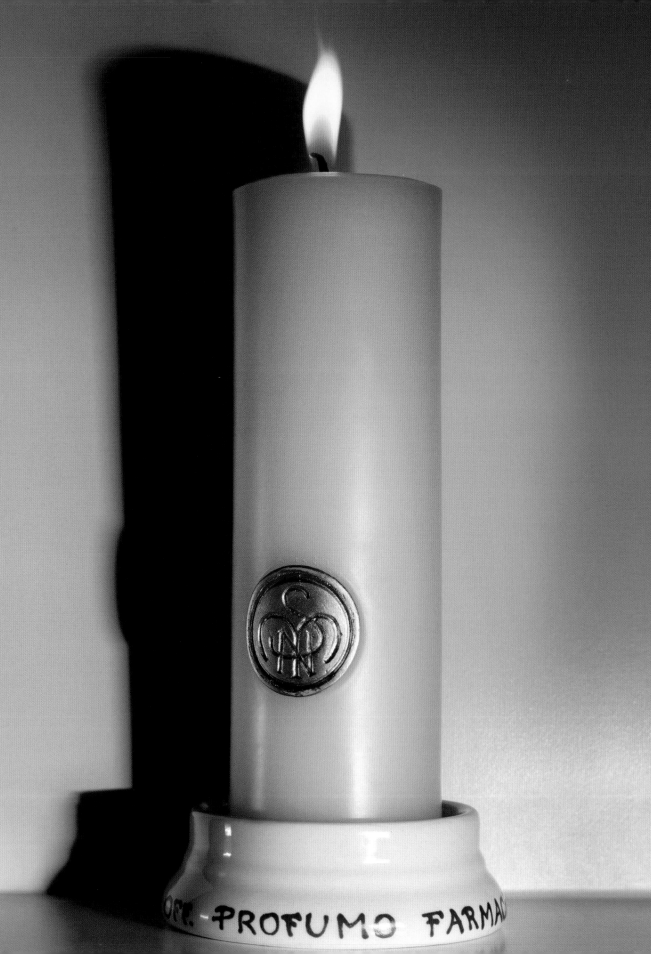

Turning Inward
This Is the Time to Focus on You

I first consulted Dr. Kenneth Y. Davis in 2001, shortly after the attacks on the World Trade Center. I had been having trouble sleeping, so a close family friend suggested that I see Dr. Davis, a chiropractor who took a holistic approach to wellness. Initially I was skeptical. I didn't see how getting an adjustment would help with my sleeplessness. When we met, Dr. Davis explained his belief that health is the result of three elements—the physical, the mental/emotional, and the spiritual—being in balance. He called this the "triangle of well-being" and said that "only 1 percent of our ills come from the physical angle" of the triangle. He told me that if I wanted to feel better, I needed to spend more time on the emotional and spiritual aspects of my being. Dr. Davis gave me many tips to help me turn my focus inward, and I continue to follow his advice today.

Practice daily meditation. This doesn't necessarily mean sitting alone and trying to empty your mind of all thoughts (few people are actually able to do this). It's about focusing your mind on a situation in front of you, consciously evaluating your choices, and then making a decision. Through this process, you become the master of your emotions instead of being reactive to circumstances. You can meditate during your morning commute or while walking around the block.

Learn the art of introspection. Before going to bed, mentally review your day from start to finish. Look at the events and situations that you were in and note what you said and did. Did you say something negative to a coworker? Did you get annoyed with the person who cut you off on the highway? You may start to notice less-than-desirable patterns in your behavior that you'll want to change.

Be in the moment. Instead of rushing to get from start to finish, slow down enough to observe what's around you. Take everything in and try to do it without tension or expectation. Realize that the present moment is all there is.

Refocus your lens. Our tendency is to focus on the negative even when there are many positive things around us. When you catch yourself falling into this pattern of negativity, interrupt it by shifting your consciousness. Think of a place that brings you joy, whistle a silly song, or picture yourself as an elephant in a pink tutu!

Breathe. Shallow breathing happens when the mind isn't present. Four to six times a day, check in with your body and how you're breathing. Stand up, put your shoulders and head back, and breathe deeply. You'll notice an immediate change in how you feel.

Keep a journal. Many people struggle to keep a journal because they worry that they won't have anything to say. Start by writing down a word or a sentence. It can be as simple as "I'm in a bad mood." If you stay with it, the sentence will eventually become a paragraph and then a page. Journaling can be a very healing exercise.

Create a sacred space. Find a space—a corner of your bedroom, the study, the bath—that's free from all distractions like ringing phones or unopened mail. Make it a place you can go to on a daily basis.

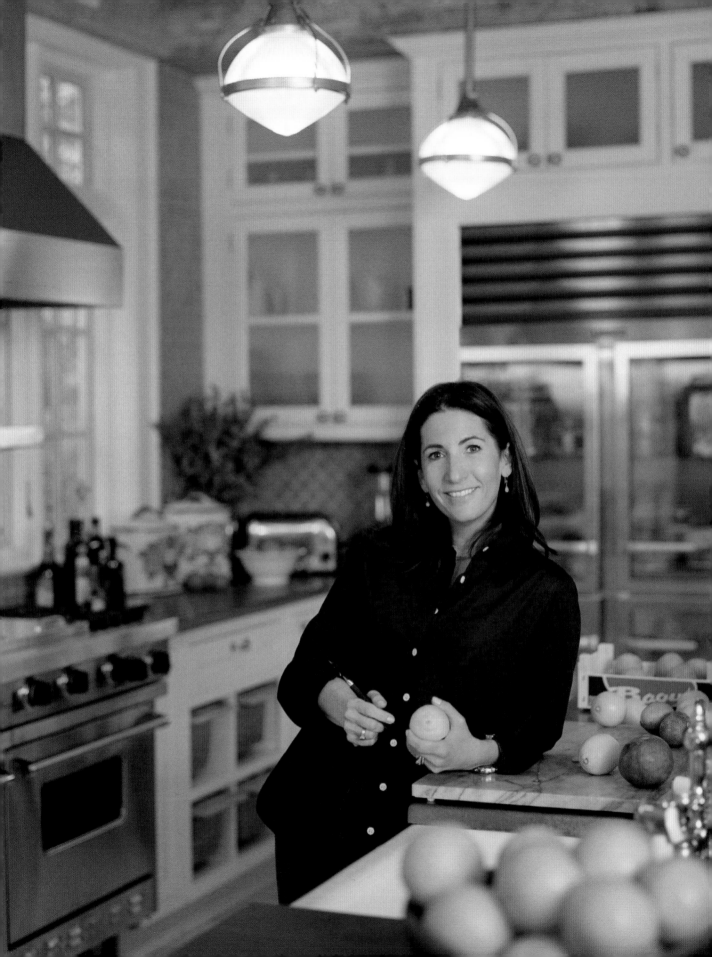

CHAPTER 7

THE REAL FOUNTAIN OF YOUTH

Eat Well and Break a Sweat

The Spanish explorer Juan Ponce de León searched in vain for the fountain of youth in the 1500s. What Ponce de León didn't realize is that you don't need healing waters to live longer. The secret to longevity is a simple combination of nutrition and exercise. I've traveled a long road in my own journey to healthy eating and balanced exercise. What I know now is that there's no such thing as a quick fix.

As a preteen I was never as thin as my friends, and I tried *anything* that promised to take the pounds off. My mother and I went on the H.O.V. diet, which involved drinking a daily mixture of honey, oil, and vinegar. It was supposed to burn fat and curb hunger. It didn't do either. Then my mother read that drinking cod-liver oil burned fat. Needless to say, that was the worst. Next, my cousin Barbara and I tried the Liquid Slender Diet. We got very skinny on this diet, but instantly gained all the weight back as soon as we ate real food. And then there was the time my pediatrician prescribed diet pills, which the pharmacist refilled without any questions. I got skinny—too skinny.

In college I was all about the Scarsdale Diet and any diet book on the bestseller list. In my twenties and thirties I tried the macrobiotic diet, the two-week juice fast, and an ionic pen that was supposed to clear the magnetic fields and extra weight in my body. It wasn't until I hit my forties that I understood and embraced the true meaning of the word *diet*.

I've finally changed my mind-set—I'm no longer striving to attain an impossible ideal. Instead of trying to be perfect, I try to be healthy. This means eating simple, wholesome foods and exercising regularly. Keep in mind that what works for me might not work for you, so approach things with an open mind. Don't beat yourself up if you get off track—just get right back on.

The Only Way to Eat

For many of us, the word *diet* has negative connotations. It means denying ourselves foods we enjoy, being hungry 24/7, and feeling guilty when we cave in to cravings. Instead, *diet* should mean eating to live, and choosing foods that taste good *and* do good too (yes, it is possible!). The right diet will not only keep you healthy but will also boost your energy and improve your looks. Common sense and moderation are the cornerstones of a healthy diet. Eat plenty of fruits, vegetables, whole grains, and lean proteins—and limit your intake of foods high in saturated fat and cholesterol. Here's how to eat your way to a healthier, more beautiful you.

Fruits and Vegetables

There are countless reasons to load up on fruits and vegetables. They're great sources of vitamins, minerals, and fiber, and are low in fat, sodium, and calories. In addition, eating produce is thought to help prevent chronic diseases. A diet that is rich in fruits and vegetables may reduce the the risk of stroke and other cardiovascular diseases, and protect against certain cancers. When shopping for your fruits and vegetables, choose a wide array of colors—everything from a red tomato to green spinach is chock-full of hidden benefits.

SIDESTEP DIET SABOTAGE

Don't let cocktail parties or nights out derail your healthy eating. Here's my game plan for staying on track: I start the day with oatmeal and an egg, go carb-free for lunch, and have a mini meal before the party. Once I'm there, I start with a glass or two of water before reaching for the red wine. I avoid all the hors d'oeuvres with the exception of the shrimp cocktail and crudités. When I get home, I eat a mini dinner of whole-grain crackers topped with low-fat cheese, tuna, or a hard-boiled egg. And if I have a sweet tooth (which happens when I drink alcohol), ricotta cheese with a sprinkling of cinnamon and vanilla does the trick.

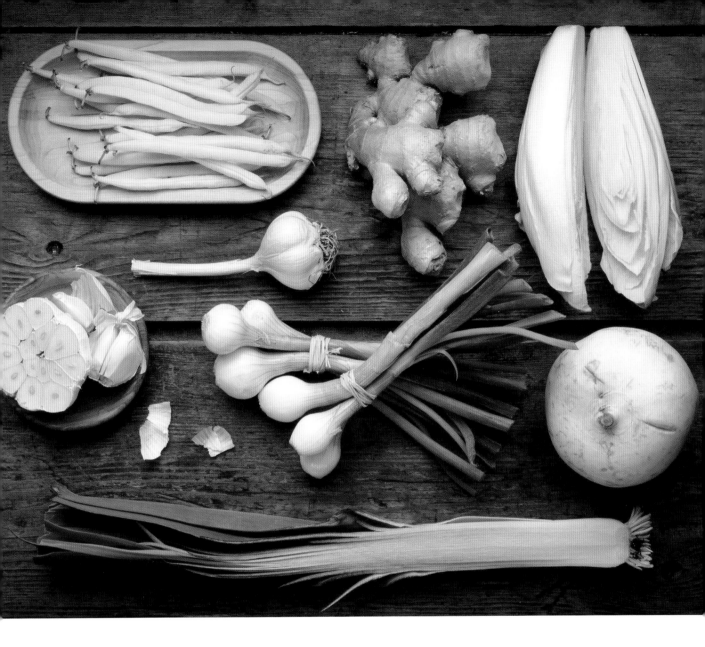

White

Vegetables like garlic, chives, scallions, and leeks contain allicin, a phytochemical that may help lower cholesterol and blood pressure, and increase the body's ability to fight off infection.

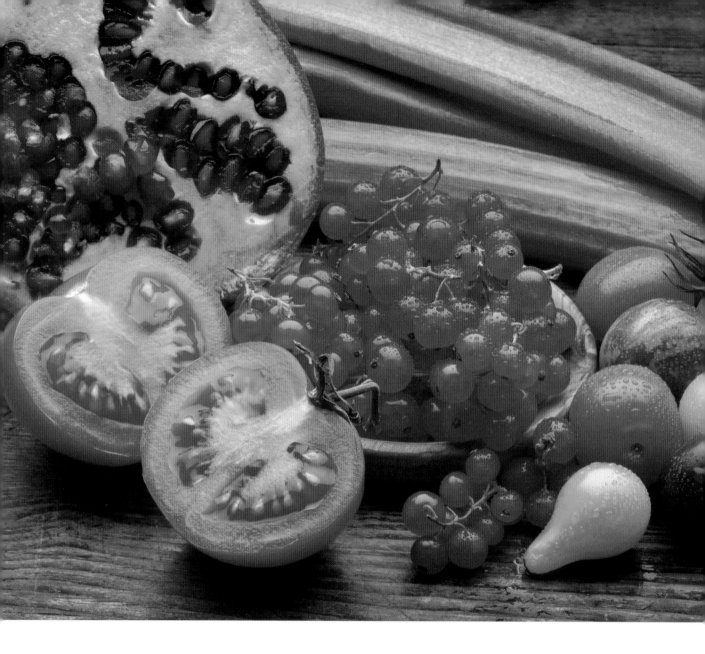

Red and Pink

Tomatoes, red and pink grapefruit, watermelon, and papaya all contain lycopene, an antioxidant that is thought to help fight heart disease and some cancers.

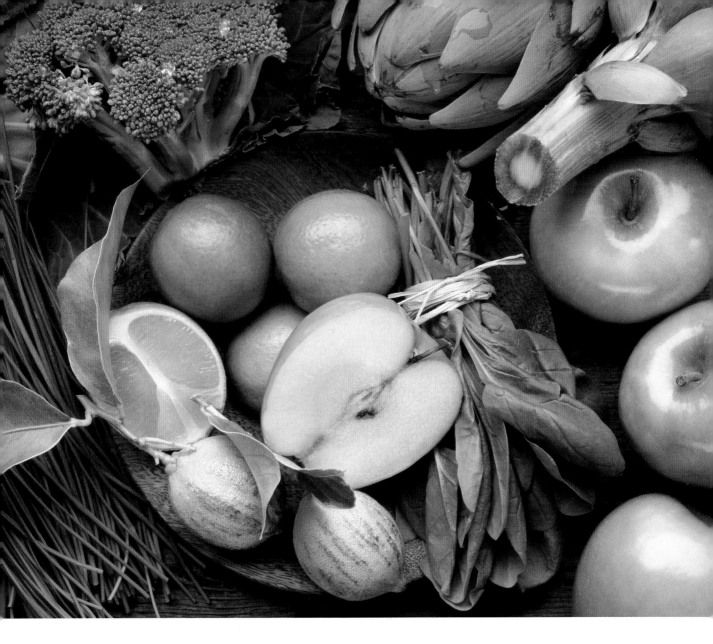

Green

Green vegetables like spinach, collard greens, kale, and broccoli are rich in fiber, have antioxidant properties, and help keep eyes healthy.

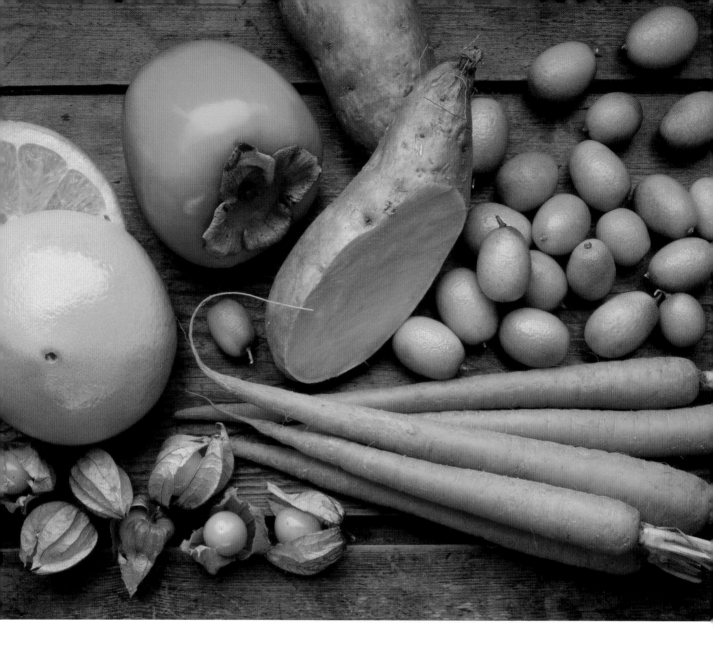

Orange and Yellow

Sweet potatoes, mangoes, and apricots all have beta-carotene, which has been shown in studies to help bolster the immune system.

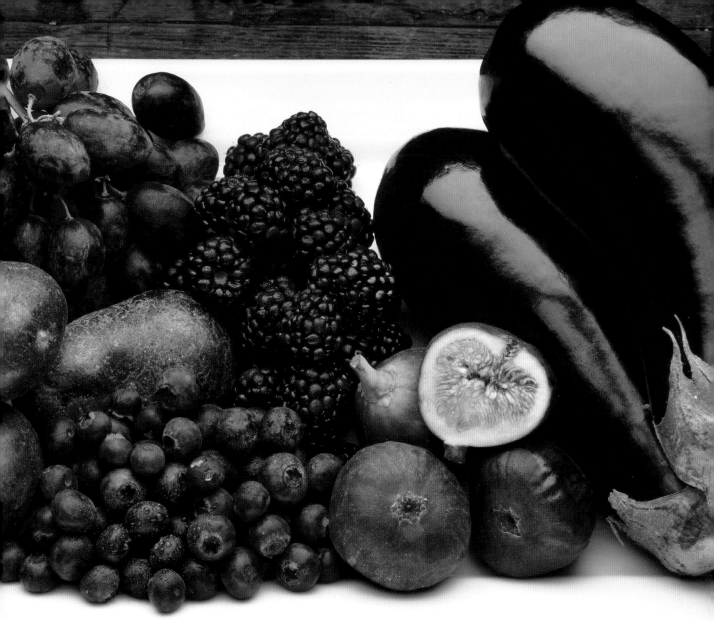

Purple and Blue

Anthocyanin, the pigment that makes blueberries and other fruits blue, is being studied for its ability to help the body defend itself against harmful carcinogens.

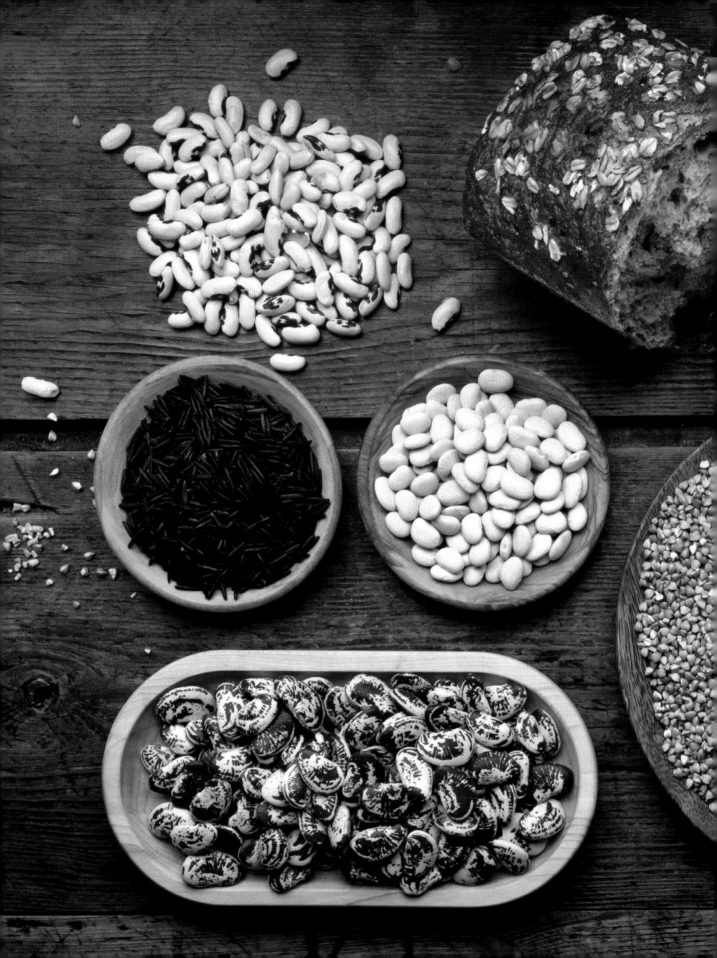

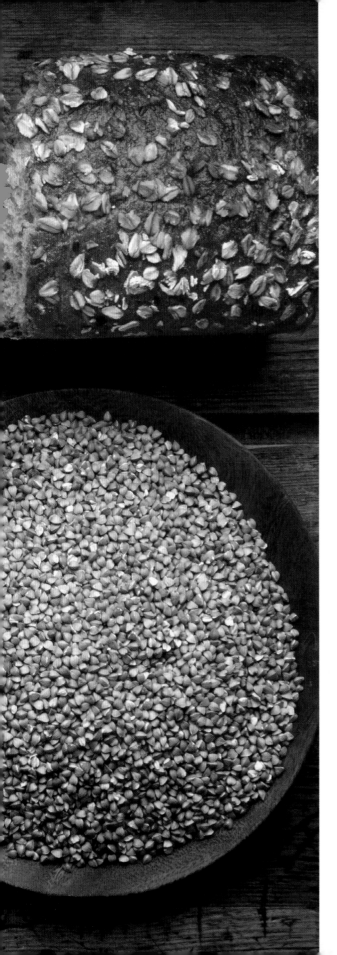

Whole Grains

Whole-grain foods are rich in fiber, which benefits the body in a number of ways. In addition to providing energy-rich starch, fiber helps reduce blood cholesterol levels and may lower risk your risk for heart disease. Fiber is also good for the digestive system; it helps keep you regular, reduces constipation, and keeps you fuller longer.

What is the difference between whole grains and refined grains? Contrary to what you might think, "refined" doesn't mean that it's better for you. Whole grains contain the entire grain kernel and are rich in fiber, nutrients, and vitamins. Examples include whole wheat, oatmeal, and brown rice. Refined grains are milled (a process that gives the grains a finer texture and longer shelf life) and do not have the fiber that the body needs. Refined grains include white flour, white bread, and white rice. The body digests whole grains much more slowly than it does refined grains. As a result, blood-sugar levels increase slowly and steadily, providing an even source of energy. Refined grains, on the other hand, cause a spike in blood-sugar levels. Since what goes up must come down, this means that you go from hyper to lethargic in a short amount of time.

A BOBBI POINTER: SMART CARBS

I believe in moderation when it comes to eating grains. On most weekdays I eat carbohydrates with breakfast and lunch, and not with dinner. On weekends I might reverse it and save the carbohydrates for dinner.

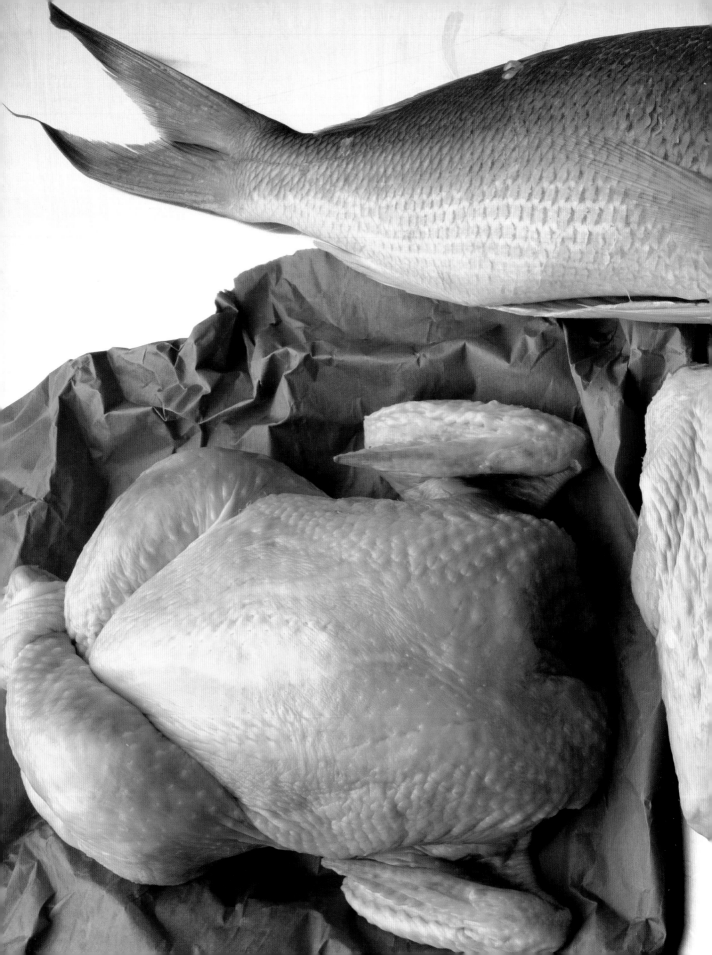

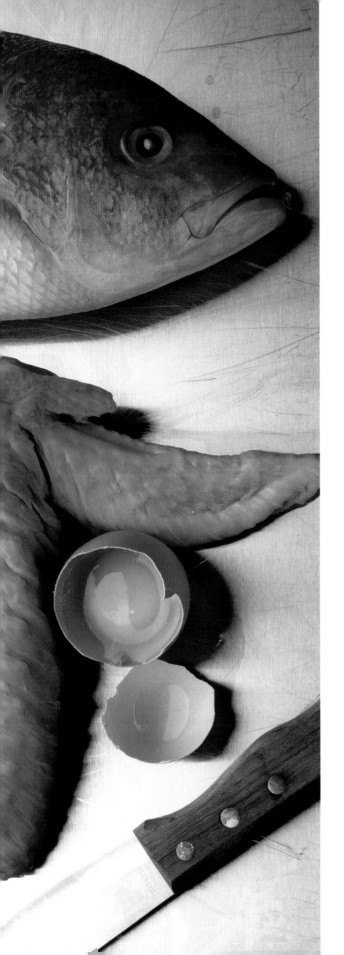

Protein

Protein, a key building block for the body, is found in poultry, fish, eggs, meat, and soy. Chicken and turkey are low in saturated fat, and fish may help reduce the risk of heart disease. After years of getting a bad rap, it turns out that eggs—when eaten in moderation—aren't nearly as bad as we thought. Studies show that the cholesterol in eggs does not increase LDL blood cholesterol levels (for more on cholesterol, see the information on fats and oils on page 154); omega-3 enriched eggs are a great way to add this nutrient to your diet. If you love red meat, eat it sparingly and choose lean cuts. Vegetarians can get their protein from soy products like tofu.

WHAT DOES ORGANIC MEAN, ANYWAY?

Browse the aisles of any grocery store today and you're likely to come across many foods bearing a sticker that says "organic." Other than cost (organic foods are typically more expensive), what's the difference between organic food and regular food? Organic food has been grown with little or no synthetic fertilizers or pesticides, and has not been treated with antibiotics or hormones. I think organic food is healthier and safer than conventionally grown food, so I do my best to buy organic—from dairy to eggs and meat.

Dairy

Milk and milk products contain good-for-your-body calcium, potassium, vitamin D, and protein. Calcium builds and maintains bone mass, and also helps reduce the risk of osteoporosis. There's no reason to avoid dairy if you're concerned about fat and calories; choose low-fat products and you'll still get your calcium and other nutrients. (I always go for organic milk). If you are lactose intolerant, take a daily calcium supplement.

Water

Staying hydrated is essential to your well-being. Water helps flush impurities out of the body, helps regulate body temperature, and carries nutrients and oxygen in the cells. Get in the habit of drinking approximately sixty-four ounces (that's eight eight-ounce glasses) of water a day. Carry a water bottle in your bag so you can hydrate easily throughout the day. To keep from getting bored, flavor your water with a splash of pomegranate juice or cranberry juice concentrate, slices of fresh lemon, lime, or cucumber, or a few sprigs of mint. I find the days I chug one to two glasses of water before my morning coffee are the days I do better with my overall water consumption.

Fats and Oils

If you've banned fat from your diet, I encourage you to consider adding it back. The body needs fat to store energy, insulate tissues, and transport fat-soluble vitamins through the blood. It's also a must for moisture in the skin. Not all fat is bad. In fact, the type of fat you eat has more of an impact on your health than the amount of fat you eat. Fat affects LDL and HDL cholesterol levels in the blood. LDL cholesterol is also known as the "bad" cholesterol because high levels are associated with an increased risk for heart attacks. HDL cholesterol, on the other hand, has been dubbed a "good" cholesterol because high levels seem to protect against heart disease.

Polyunsaturated and monounsaturated fats in your diet can help reduce LDL cholesterol levels and decrease the risk for heart disease. Polyunsaturated fats are found in safflower, corn, and canola oils, and fish like salmon and mackerel. Monounsaturated fats are present in canola, olive, and peanut oils. Avoid foods high in saturated fats (found in all junk food) because they increase LDL cholesterol levels.

BOBBI POINTER: 10 TIPS FOR HEALTHY EATING

◆

I've learned to make the right choices 90 percent of the time. The remaining 10 percent is reserved for times when it's really worth it—I can never turn down my aunt Alice's toffee squares or the French fries at Balthazar, a restaurant in New York City, and I don't worry about what I eat when I travel to Paris or Italy.

Here are my strategies for healthy eating:

1. Read ingredient labels to be a well-informed eater. Pass on processed, chemical-laden food.
2. Choose whole grains over white flour.
3. Enjoy lots of fresh greens and fruits.
4. Load up on proteins like chicken, fish, and beans. Red meat is OK on occasion.
5. Drink lots of water. In addition to hydrating, water transports nutrients, flushes out toxins, and gives you lots of energy.
6. Eat every two to three hours. Don't let yourself get ravenous.
7. Treats like red wine, dark chocolate, and raw almonds are OK in small amounts.
8. Take your vitamins.
9. Always strive for better, not perfect.
10. And most important, remember that calories do count. Portion control is everything.

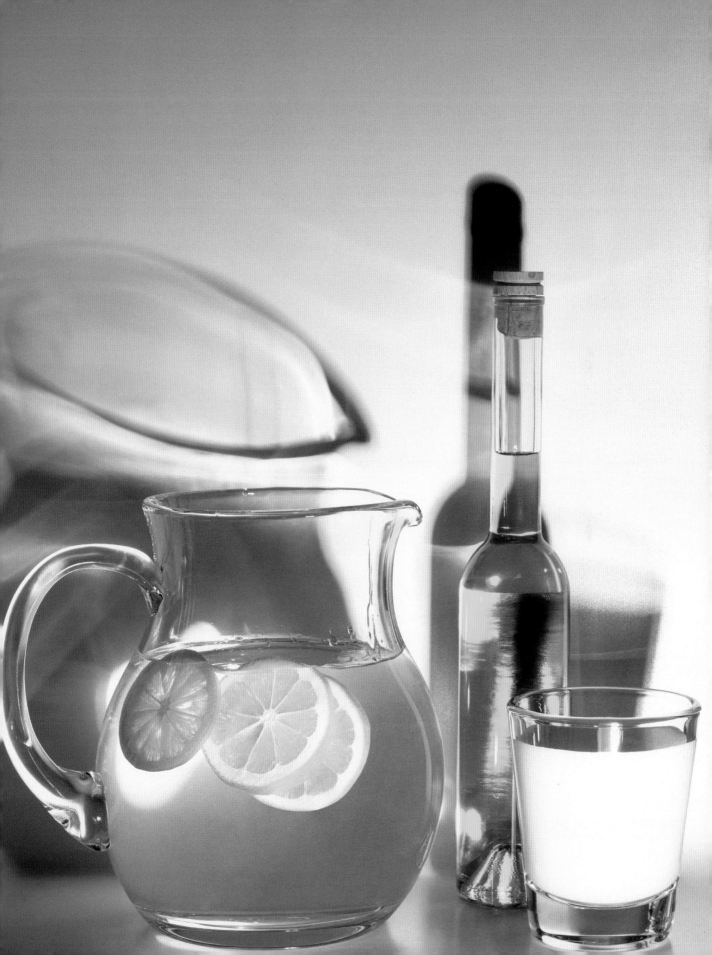

Bobbi's Favorite Meals

Breakfast I love slow-cooked Irish oatmeal (you can make it the night before and reheat it the following morning). I load up on calcium with plain Greek yogurt flavored with cinnamon and slivers of roasted almonds. And I swear by egg-white omelets with seven-grain toast.

Lunch When lunch rolls around, I never get tired of what I call "chopped kitchen salad." It's easy to make and so satisfying. In a big bowl I toss together: alfalfa sprouts, asparagus, baby arugula, bok choy, green beans, mushrooms, tomatoes, cooked egg whites, tuna or chicken, and low-fat cheese. If you're especially hungry, supplement your salad with a mini serving of brown rice or whole-grain bread.

Instead of store-bought dressing, I top my salad with my own homemade dressing. To make it, combine cold-pressed olive oil, a splash of balsamic vinegar, Dijon mustard, fresh chopped garlic, kosher salt, and cracked black pepper. Don't worry about exact measurements for the ingredients—go by taste.

Dinner After a long day at work, there's nothing more comforting for dinner than a steaming bowl of soup. In a blender, combine 2 cans of organic chicken broth, 2 to 3 cups of cooked broccoli or zucchini, 1/2 to 1 cup frozen organic peas, kosher salt, and cracked black pepper; blend until smooth. Transfer the mixture to a pot and bring it to a boil over medium heat. Top individual soup bowls with a dollop of plain Greek yogurt or cottage cheese and a sprinkling of chopped fresh chives. I'll also have a bit of fish or chicken and a tiny portion of spelt pasta. And, of course, a glass of red wine.

Dessert I satisfy my sweet tooth with plain Greek yogurt (as you can see, it's incredibly versatile) topped with chocolate protein powder, or low-fat ricotta cheese sweetened with maple syrup and cinnamon. Fresh fruit topped with homemade whipped cream or vanilla yogurt is another filling dessert.

THE SKINNY ON SWEETENERS

As a mom, I'd rather see my kids eat sugar than artificial sweeteners; I'm most happy to see them eat fruit. But if you're trying to lose weight, you have to keep your sugar intake under control. If you must go the artificial route, use Splenda in moderation (it's a source of some controversy because it's a synthetic compound). Stevia is another option, but I don't love how it tastes. Stay away from diet soda and diet drink mixes that contain aspartame.

How to Detox After Overindulging

David Kirsch, a New York–based fitness guru, has helped countless stars get into enviable shape. I met David five years ago at an industry event and instantly fell in love with his approach to diet and exercise. David's as hard core as it gets—he's taught me how to clean up my diet and has pushed me physically to places I never thought I could go. On the occasions when I fall off the wellness wagon, I clean up my act by following David's no-nonsense advice:

• No matter how bad you feel, get your butt out of bed and start moving around. The worst thing you can do is to lie under the covers and bemoan your state and your growing, pounding hangover.

• Start hydrating immediately. Water (plain or with a vitamin mineral powder) is great. Herbal tea will do as well.

• Now that you're up and moving (sort of), start trying to work up a bit of a sweat—the more you are capable of doing, the better, even if it's just a power walk down to the mailbox, a power walk with man's best friend, or if you're really brave, a stint on the elliptical machine that has been collecting dust and doubling as one of your closets.

• The more you sweat, the more you'll be getting rid of those nasty toxins. You'll know when you start smelling the cocktails you were drinking the night before.

• If it was the trip to the local pizzeria or donut shop that has you blue, then you have probably awakened to what I have been known to call "carb face," and again, there's nothing like a good sweat to shed the extra weight and bloat.

• Often I tell my clients to start the day with a protein shake (a great way to fuel up on the run without weighing you down). For added energy, mix up some vitamin and mineral powder and you are "off to the races."

• If you're stuck at home, do a circuit of the following exercises, fifteen to twenty repetitions each without rest in between. If you survive the first circuit, try to challenge yourself and do it again. In this case my mantra is "if some is good, more is definitely better": plié squats, alternate reverse lunges, push-ups with hip extension, double crunches, and shadow boxing (for about 1 minute). That covers the entire body and should help you feel more human again and light of foot.

• As far as eating, don't make the mistake of starving yourself in response to last night's overindulgence. The best thing is to eat clean, light salads and proteins like chicken, fish, and egg whites. If you are a vegetarian, then stick to tofu.

• If it was alcohol that got the better of you, then you'll be craving something "nice and greasy." Stay away from the cheeseburgers and fries! If it's comfort food you are seeking and your body is craving, then I would try some Irish oatmeal to start the day. Follow that up with an egg-white omelet with spinach and shiitake mushrooms and turkey bacon.

My Fitness Epiphany

Growing up, I was never very athletic. I tried ballet and clearly wasn't built for it. Instead of running around and climbing trees like the other kids, I spent my time doing arts and crafts. In high school, I did everything I could to avoid gym class. I hated running and I didn't care much for field hockey (plus, the outfits we had to wear were just plain embarrassing). My mother wrote me many notes excusing me from gym class over the course of those four years. In college I learned how to diet my way to thin and never thought of exercise.

It wasn't until I graduated from college that I had my fitness epiphany. I joined a gym and almost instantly saw the difference. I felt better, got stronger, and was able to eat more. I was hooked. When I was a young, starving makeup artist in New York, I took high-impact aerobics classes. I remember working out next to Madonna when she was an up-and-coming star. *Flash Dance* was all the rage, so I had workout outfits inspired by Jennifer Beals' look in the movie. I wore knit leggings scrunched just so around my ankles and cut the neck off a stretched and worn-out black sweatshirt so it would fall off my shoulder. I ended up doing Jennifer's makeup years later when I was an established makeup artist and she laughed when I told her my story.

I was twenty-five when I realized the importance of weight training. I remember looking down at my legs and noticing that things looked a little looser and less toned. I immediately started a weight routine and thankfully, it worked (and still does today). My outlook on exercise really evolved when I was in my thirties and forties. I learned how important it is to work on core strength and flexibility, so I started taking classes in Pilates and the Lotte Berk Method (which is based on a dancer's workout). My fitness routine now is a combination of workouts on the elliptical machine (it's kind on my joints), speed walking (I wear a pedometer to track the number of steps I've taken and usually meet my goal of 10,000 steps by going on an hour walk with my girlfriends), running, spinning, yoga, and weights.

Need Reasons to Get Moving?

You'll live longer and look better. The benefits of exercise go far beyond losing weight. Exercising regularly can help stave off many of the negative effects that aging has on the body—and fit women age beautifully. Experts agree that even half an hour of exercise a day makes a difference, so stop making excuses and break a sweat now.

Exercise is good for your heart and lungs. Working out helps reduce your risk for heart disease. It decreases LDL (bad cholesterol) levels and increases HDL (good cholesterol) levels in the blood. In addition, exercising can help prevent the onset of high blood pressure, which is good news for those with a family history of hypertension. If your blood pressure is already on the high end, exercise can help lower it. Lungs reap the benefit of consistent aerobic activity too; they're better able to take in oxygen, which in turn nourishes the body's cells.

Exercise builds up your bones and muscles. As it ages, the body loses both bone density and muscle mass. The good news is that strength training and weight-bearing exercises can actually help slow down and reverse this process. Studies show that weight training and resistance work protect existing bone and may even help build new bone (a key benefit for menopausal and postmenopausal women, who are susceptible to osteoporosis, a weakening of the bones). These exercises also help decrease the loss of lean muscle tissue and replace lost muscle tissue. Strong bones and muscles improve both your balance and your coordination, reducing the risk of falls and painful breaks.

Exercise helps keep your weight in check. Math has never been my forte, but this is a simple equation that makes sense. If you want to lose weight, you need to burn more calories than you consume. As I mentioned above, exercise helps build muscle—and muscle burns more calories than fat (even when you're resting). Maintaining a healthy weight takes pressure off your bones and joints, which can help prevent arthritis.

Exercise helps prevent disease. Regular exercise combined with a healthy diet can help prevent and manage type 2 diabetes (also known as adult-onset diabetes), a condition that affects the body's ability to metabolize sugar properly. Exercise has also been shown to help lower the risk for certain types of cancer like colon cancer, cancer of the uterine lining, and breast cancer.

Exercise cheers you up. It's no coincidence that people who work out are generally more relaxed than those who don't. When I skip a day or two of exercise I immediately see a difference in my mood and how I react to stress around me. What's the reason? Working out stimulates the production of endorphins, neurotransmitters that enhance your mood and provide natural pain relief.

Exercise helps you get your Z's. Moderate exercise a few hours before bedtime can help rid your body of excess stress and tension—and get you ready for bed.

A BOBBI POINTER: MUSIC THAT GETS ME GOING

1. "Hot in Here" Nelly
2. "Satisfaction" The Rolling Stones
3. "The Way You Move" OutKast
4. "Think" Aretha Franklin
5. "With or Without You" U2
6. "Lose Yourself" Eminem
7. "We Will Rock You" Queen
8. "Born to Run" Bruce Springsteen
9. "Smooth" Carlos Santana
10. *Saturday Night Fever* (the whole album)

THE TALK TEST

How do you know if you're pushing yourself enough during your workout? Try talking. If you're able to carry on a conversation easily, the intensity level of your workout is light to moderate. If you get winded trying to speak a full sentence, you're exercising vigorously. Just remember, you have to sweat to make changes!

How to Make Exercise Work for You

There is no such thing as a one-size-fits-all fitness program. We are all built differently, so a regimen that works for your coworker or your friend won't necessarily work for you. Do anything—just do it daily. Before lacing up your sneakers, take a moment to ask yourself some key questions. Your answers will help you decide what kind of exercises you should be doing.

What's your end goal?

Do you want to drop a few dress sizes, get six-pack abs, or run a race? Once you're clear on the goal, break it down into short-term and long-term achievements. A challenge is much less intimidating and easier to take on when you look at it in increments.

What are your physical strengths and weaknesses?

If you're able to go for miles on the treadmill but aren't very toned, you may want to incorporate weight lifting into your workouts. Cross training like this not only keeps you from getting bored, but it also helps reduce the chances that you'll overuse or injure one muscle or joint.

What activities do you enjoy?

Choose exercises that complement your lifestyle. For example, if you love to bike you'll most likely enjoy a spinning class. Remember, anything that increases your pulse makes a difference.

Are you a people person or do you enjoy solo time?

If you feel most inspired when you're surrounded by people, try a group class at a gym. On the other hand, if you often seek time alone, you may prefer working out at home or on the machines at the gym (an iPod with upbeat music will keep you working longer).

Schedule your workouts for the week and commit to them in the same way that you commit to work meetings or plans with friends and family. An exercise routine is easier to stick to when the time is already accounted for on your calendar. And since life sometimes throws curveballs, cut yourself a break when you don't feel well or when you feel like you're burning the candle on both ends. A day or two off from exercising isn't the end of the world, and you'll probably come back to your workouts with more energy and a better attitude.

A Three-Pronged Approach to Fitness

Fitness is a combination of three elements: aerobic fitness, muscular fitness, and flexibility. When you're **aerobically fit**, your body is more efficient at converting oxygen into energy. This means that you can work out at a higher intensity for a longer period of time. Examples of aerobic activity include running, bicycling, swimming, kickboxing, and step class. When you're **muscularly fit**, it shows both inside and out—muscles are stronger and your body is more toned. To improve your muscular fitness, lift weights (whether you use weight machines or free weights is a matter of personal preference) or try exercises like push-ups and lunges. Work on your **flexibility** to increase your range of motion and help decrease both muscle soreness and exercise-related injures. Yoga and Pilates are both good ways to get more limber.

Just Say "Om"

Molly Fox's fitness classes were all the rage when I was in my twenties. She was high-energy, incredibly intense, and in some ways a little intimidating. When I reconnected with Molly recently to ask her to share her fitness expertise in this chapter, I was instantly taken by her now Zenlike energy. Her secret? Her fitness regimen has evolved from intense aerobics to intense yoga. On pages 162–163, Molly shares her tips for finding the best yoga practice for you.

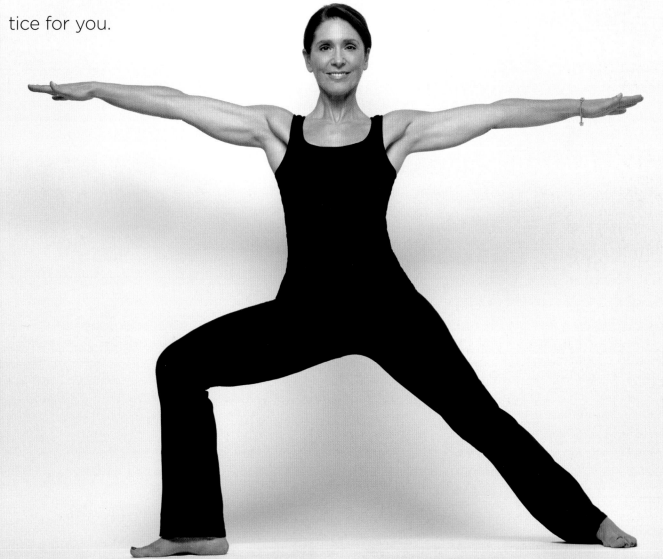

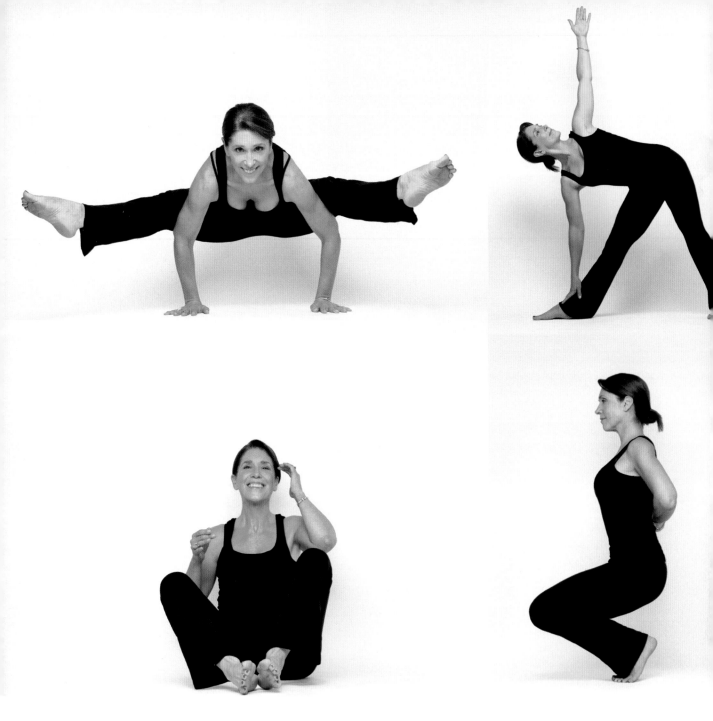

Fitness-Oriented Yoga If you want to sweat, tone up, and get stronger, try Vinyasa Yoga, Ashtanga Yoga, Power Yoga, Forrest Yoga, Jivamukti Yoga, Budakon (blend of yoga, meditation, and martial arts), or Bikram Yoga (practiced in a room heated over 100 degrees). Most of these include push-ups, strong leg poses, abdominal work, and core work to strengthen your posture.

Stress Management, Relaxation, and Revujenation If you want to reduce your stress levels, let go of tension, increase your inner sensitivity, increase your flexibility, and just feel better, try Restorative Yoga, Kripalu Yoga, Intregal Yoga, or Gentle Yoga. These classes may focus on holding gentle poses longer, focusing on your breath and letting go of tension. Some may have more of a spiritual bent which may include chanting.

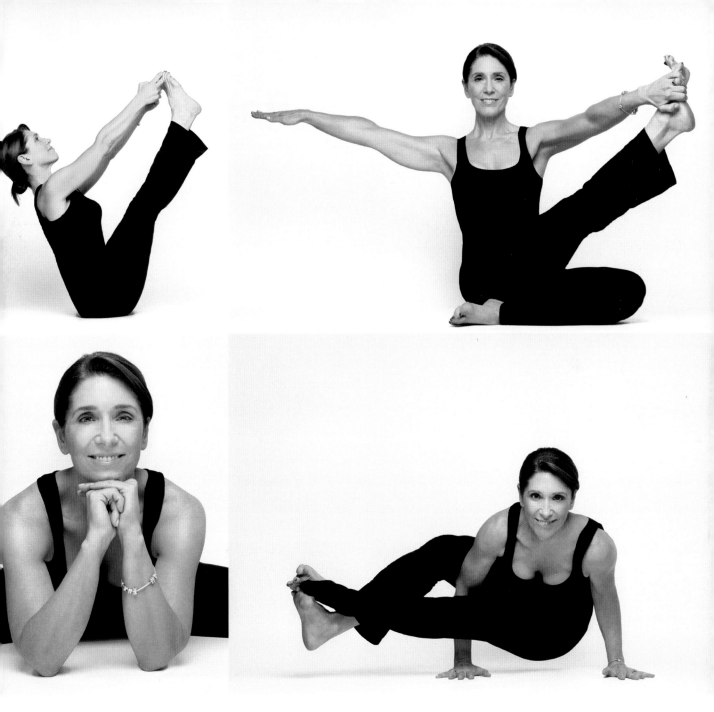

Therapeutic Yoga Also a workout, this is a good choice if you want to heal injuries, improve your posture, increase your breath capacity, reduce stress, and open your heart. Iyengar Yoga, Anusara Yoga, and Viniyoga provide alignment and core strengthening. Iyengar is known for using props, holding poses longer, and creating strength and freedom in your poses. Anusara Yoga is known for a system of principles of alignment and for exploring the idea of opening your heart for increased joy and spiritual development. Viniyoga focuses on alignment from the inside out. Practicing moving with your breath will result in deeper breath and freer movements, strength, and flexibility, and will increase the body/mind connection.

Case Study
Deborah Medeiros-Baker

A 12-WEEK NUTRITION AND FITNESS MAKEOVER

Deborah: "When I look in the mirror, I see a buildup of time. I don't think I look bad for fifty, but I'm disappointed that I'm not in better shape. When I was younger, people called me Twiggy. I exercised regularly as a young adult, but let exercise fall by the wayside when I had babies. Trying to balance family and work, it was easy to let exercise go. Working as a freelance stylist, I keep very irregular hours and don't have a set eating schedule. When I'm stressed, I indulge in late-night snacks.

"I would like to get dressed without worrying about concealing my flaws. I have a closet filled with shapewear that I'd like to get rid of! My body has changed and high cholesterol runs in my family, so I'd like to learn how to eat right for my body. I'm not trying to go back to 1985. I just want to do better with what I have."

Bobbi: I took Deborah to Platinum Fitness in New Jersey and teamed her up with Rich Fitter, a nutritionist, and Monica Trentin, a trainer. They had twelve weeks to whip Deborah into shape and their goal was to reduce Deborah's body fat by 8 percent.

Rich's plan: "Deborah has to change the way she looks at food. A lot of women think that they can't eat if they want to lose weight. Sixty-five percent of the calories we consume are used by the body for basic bodily processes. Most women who diet don't consume enough calories to satisfy this need. They end up losing water weight and muscle and bone density, but no fat.

"When you're trying to change your diet, it's important to be mindful of what you eat. Keep a written log of your meals to see what your daily patterns are. You'll probably have foods that you enjoy more than others. Instead of cutting these foods out I believe in figuring out how to structure a diet so that it can still accommodate your favorites.

"Deborah's program is all about planning ahead. If Deborah knows she's going to be on a shoot with unhealthy food options, she needs to plan for it by packing her meals the night before. Studies show that it takes about three weeks to turn a new behavior into a habit, so Deborah may initially have a hard time breaking her old ways."

Monica's plan: "Deborah wants to improve her overall fitness and energy levels. She'd like to tone up her abdominal area and increase her flexibility. Her exercise regimen calls for a mix of thirty-minute cardio sessions four days a week and two days of strength training.

"I can't say enough to emphasize the importance of strength training and working the body from the core out. The biggest misconception women have about lifting weights is that it will make them big. I've actually had clients tell me that they have to go on a diet before they start weight training.

"Deborah's challenge will be to make the time to exercise. Since she doesn't have set office hours, it's harder for her to keep herself on a schedule. My advice for Deborah is twofold: to take it a week at a time, and to map out her exercise plans for that particular week. And if she misses a planned workout, rather than stressing out about it, she's going to look to see where else in the week she can fit it in."

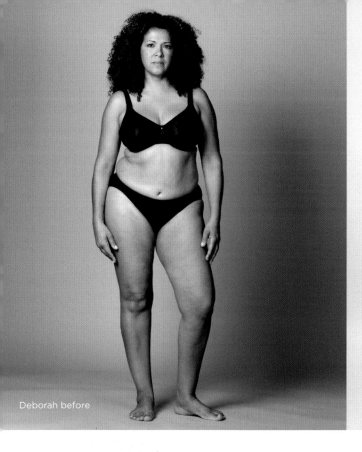

Deborah before

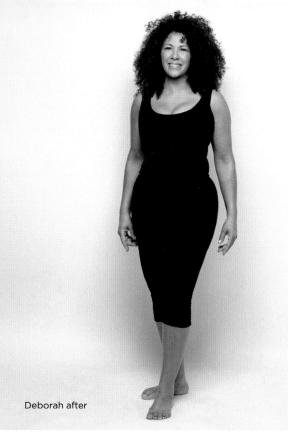

Deborah after

PROGRESS: "This program has forced me to be conscious of how I use the time in my day, and as a result, it's actually helped me with my overall time management. Believe it or not, one of my other challenges has been making sure that I eat small meals every few hours—I actually have to remind myself to eat! Even though I'm only halfway through the program, I already see and feel the improvements. I love how I feel after working out…it's almost euphoric. I'm not as stressed as I used to be and instead of seeking comfort in food, I've learned to find comfort in other ways—like making a cup of tea or reading a book I love. My pants are fitting looser and buttons don't pull the way they used to. I can breathe again. I like the progress I'm making and I don't want to set myself back. So when I go out with friends now, I say no to a martini and instead I'll sip a glass of red wine and some water."

RESULTS: "This program was the jump start I needed. At first I was shocked at how little weight I lost, but I learned that going down in fat percentage is far more important than the pounds you drop. My biggest challenges during the three-month period were scheduling my time (because my schedule is so erratic) and eating the right things frequently throughout the day. I now understand that you can't starve your body; otherwise it goes into survival mode and starts to store and build up fat. Working out helped me beat my late-night cravings.

"A lot of times I would stop myself from reaching for a cookie or piece of chocolate because it didn't seem worth it. My biggest tip for anyone who wants to get healthier? Just do it. Start something, anything, even if it's walking in the park. Get your friends involved. Instead of meeting for drinks or talking on the phone, make plans to catch up at the gym."

Body Fat % Before: 37.2% Body Fat % After: 31.9%
Lean Body Mass Before: 112.098 lbs.
Lean Body Mass After: 119.175 lbs.

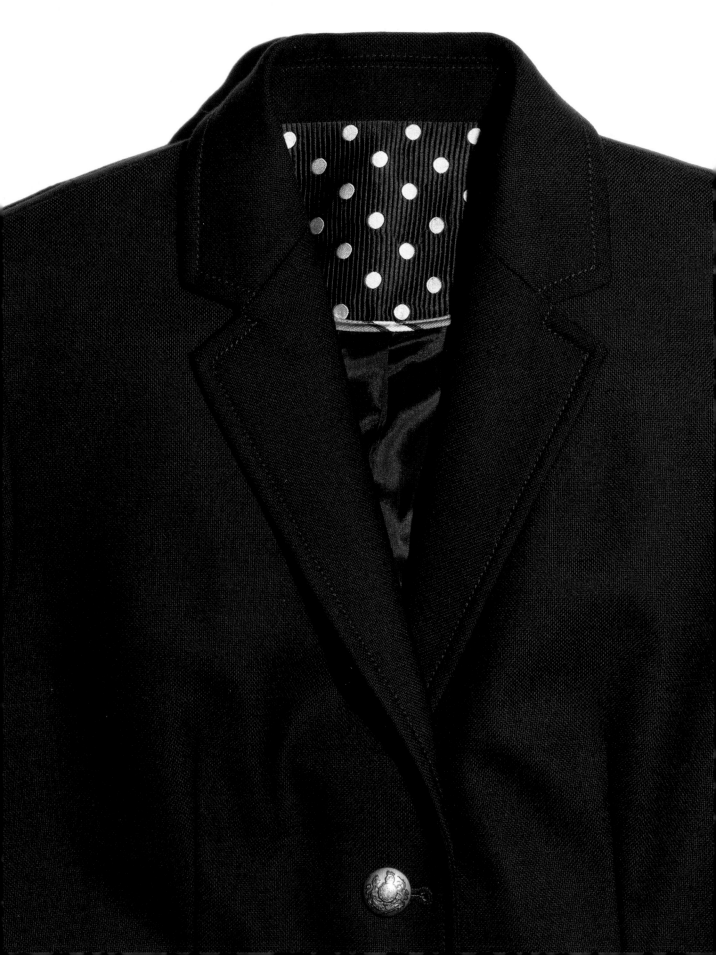

CHAPTER 8

HEAD-TO-TOE MAKEOVERS

Fresh Ways to Modernize Your Look

I've been very fortunate to be around many talented people in the beauty and fashion business for so many years. From stylists and hairdressers to designers and magazine editors, they are the ones who know what works. What I've learned from them is that trendy, funky looks work for a select few—and classic, clean looks are the best way to go for the rest of us. You don't have to spend a lot of money to have great style. In fact, my favorite looks are those that mix one great piece with less expensive items. Invest in a good suit, shoes, or handbag—something that is so classic that you'll have it five to ten years from now—and pair it with inexpensive items that you can update each season. Simple, fitted clothes (ones that are not too tight or too big) will always work (for more information, see Chapter 5). Think modern and classic. Think updated and flattering. Just make it work for your style. Start by observing women you admire to see what works. Cut out pictures from magazines for inspiration and tips. And remember, even one update can make all the difference. Take a look at the dramatic results achieved by the women in this chapter.

Abby Cooperberg

What We Did Abby is in phenomenal shape (she takes tons of spinning classes), but you don't see that because she gets lost in clothes that are too big for her. I knew that just putting her in a form-fitting outfit would make a huge difference. Since her style is simple, I picked a fitted crewneck shirt, a black blazer, flared jeans, and heels. When you wear a longer jean with a slight flare it makes you look taller. And the pointy shoes are hip. Abby's hair was about 70 percent gray, so we used a combination of beigey blonde highlights and warm chestnut lowlights to warm her up. We gave her a very natural makeup look, but made sure it was strong enough to liven up her face. Small touches like dark brown eyeliner, pale pink cream blush, and a buff-colored lip gloss made a big difference.

Before "In general, I don't feel like I look that bad, but I know that I don't look my best. My everyday look is very casual and I don't get dressed up unless it's for a really big occasion. I don't wear much makeup and I've noticed lately that my eyes have been looking tired. I have naturally curly hair and some highlights. I'm not great at upkeep and I don't regularly get my hair cut or colored. In terms of clothing, I normally wear jeans and loose-fitting tops that I can layer. Nothing too snug. I generally wear sneakers, flats, or boots with a low heel—never high heels. This is what I'm comfortable in."

After "I was quite surprised by how different I looked. My hair was styled straight, which I wasn't comfortable with because I think straight hair makes my face look longer. I liked the makeup because it looked natural and it was still within what was reasonable for me. The long jeans and bronze pumps looked amazing in the picture, but I didn't find them practical for everyday wear. While many of the elements of the makeover weren't realistic for me, I enjoyed the experience because it showed me how much better I can look with a little extra effort."

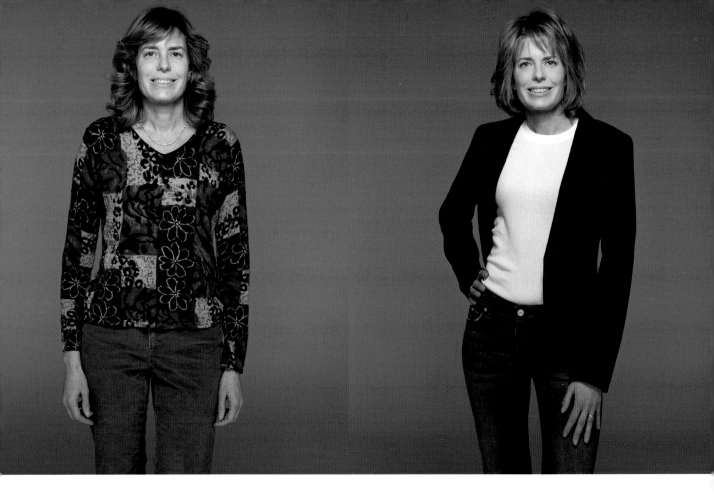

Abby's Tips Makeovers are a great way to try something new and you can adapt the elements that work for you. I now style my hair somewhere in between straight and curly, and that's made a big difference.

Don't wait for a special occasion to get dressed up. Depending on my mood now, I'll spend a bit more time to dress less casually.

You don't need to wear a face full of makeup to look better. It's about knowing what looks great on you. For me, it's eyeliner, mascara, and a bit of blush.

I think maintaining good health is the secret to aging well. I try to exercise three times a week. On days when I can't work out, I stretch at home for about twenty minutes.

Debby Fitzgerald

What We Did I've known Debby for over a decade (since our kids were in pre-kindergarten). Her look has pretty much stayed the same over the years, and she was long overdue for an update. Our goal was to give her a more modern look without looking trendy.

Debby doesn't usually wear a lot of makeup, so we kept her look natural with a tinted moisturizing balm and natural bronzing powder to warm up her skin. To make her beautiful blue eyes pop, we lined her eyes with navy eye shadow. Petal pink lip pencil and clear gloss on her lips completed the look. We gave Debby's hair caramel highlights to brighten up her face. To freshen up her cut, we shortened the back and texturized the front (which also added fullness). For the finishing touch, we dressed Debby in body-flattering clothes: a simple white top, a fitted velvet blazer, and long stylish jeans. The look was a bit hip, but still subtle. It's amazing how the smallest changes can make such a big difference.

Before "I have a pretty busy life—I work and I have kids—so I've stuck to the same routine for a long time now. I have a very basic beauty regimen: I wash and condition my hair, moisturize my face, and put on a bit of blush and mascara. In terms of my clothing, I like to be comfortable and I have to be able to move around. I usually wear suits at work and sweaters and pants at home. I feel like I'm in a rut. I'd like to look a little fresher and want something that will jazz me up a bit."

After "I thought I looked fresher, more relaxed, and sparkly. Even though I had more makeup on than I normally wear, I still looked natural, which was important to me. My skin felt really good—like it was breathing more—and I think it had to do with the eye cream and rich face cream that was applied before the makeup. The biggest change for me was definitely the hair. The highlights, which looked like the golden highlights I naturally had when I was younger, really brightened me up. My outfit was very stylish and about twenty-five years ahead of where I usually dress! The jeans were a big departure from the pants I own. The shoes looked great, but I don't see myself wearing them on a regular basis."

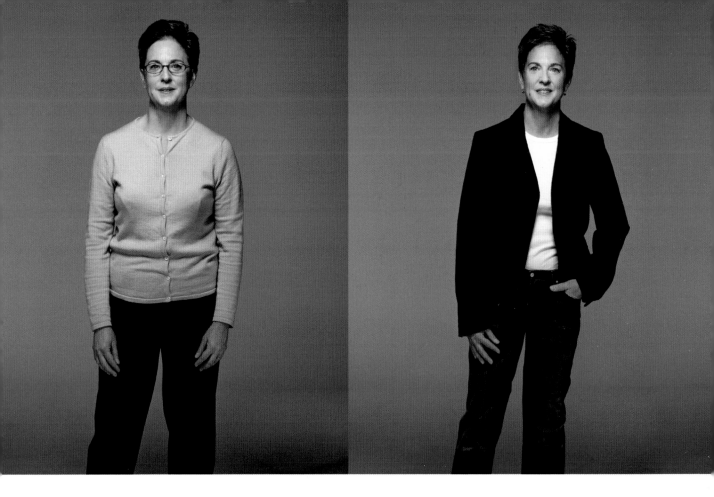

Debby's Tips Taking good, consistent care of your skin is so important. The area around my eyes looks and feels much fresher since I added an eye cream to my daily routine. Lips get thinner and less defined with age, so I've learned that lining them is a good way to add back some definition and fullness.

Don't be afraid to experiment when you go shopping. Now I'm more open to trying different designers to see if there are ones that are more flattering for my body type. (Good tip: take your teenage daughter shopping!)

You're far from over when you hit forty or fifty. In fact, this is just the beginning for me—I feel like it's finally my time to be my most active, most engaged, and most vital.

Linda Fann

What We Did Linda is a perfect example of someone who needs only a little tweaking to see big results. She has great style, so we didn't want to change it—we just wanted to make the slightest tweaks, like putting her in a pair of jeans that's one size smaller (and a lot hipper) and going for a more tailored look on top with a cashmere sweater and slim-cut blazer. In keeping with Linda's less-is-more approach, we used just the essentials on her face: a tinted moisturizer that was sheer enough to let her freckles show through, a stick foundation to cover her dark circles and the sunspot that was bothering her, a sheer brownish-pink lip tint, and some mascara. She wanted to keep her hair "wash and go," so we trimmed two inches off to get rid of the weight at the ends.

Before "I tend to be really minimal when it comes to my physical appearance. Between juggling my kids and working, I have never had the luxury of spending a lot of time on myself, so I try to pick things that are simple and easy to deal with. I don't get my hair done a lot and I don't dye it. In terms of clothing, I opt for pantsuits for work and jeans and sweaters on the weekends. My beauty routine is limited to face wash, moisturizer, and some eye cream. I have a spot on my face which seems to have gotten bigger and I would like to make it less prominent."

After "Considering that I didn't want to do this makeover when Bobbi first approached me, I have to say that the experience was much better than I thought it would be. Everyone—from Bobbi to the hairdresser to the stylist—was very conscious of doing things within my comfort level. This makeover was very much about a personal fit and not about 'we think you should wear this, this, and this.'"

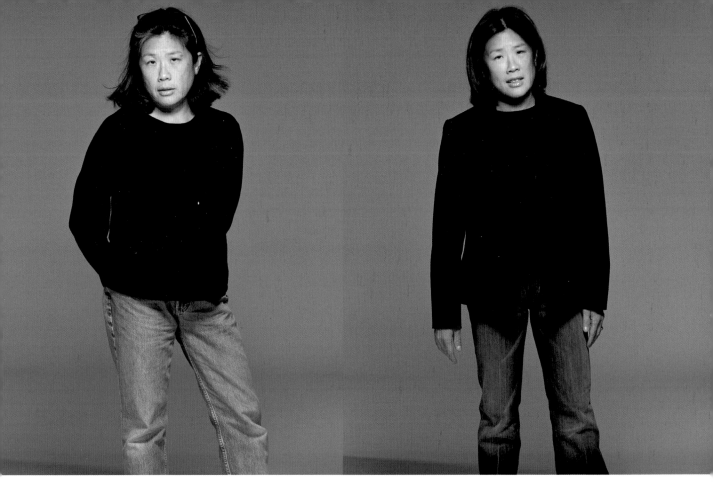

Linda's Tips A sleek blazer is a great wardrobe staple. Depending on what you pair it with, it can go easily from weekday to weekend.

My shoulder-length hair can get bulky, and I've learned that taking weight off the ends is the trick to making it a wash-and-go hairdo.

Beauty is having your own look and style. It's not about subscribing to conventional forms of beauty— it's doing what you're comfortable with.

Linda Berkovic

What We Did Linda was hiding in a big outfit, so our goal was to teach her that you don't have to be skinny to wear the right clothes. We put her in body-smoothing undergarments and showed her how the right pants could actually make her legs look long and thin. (She was making the common fashion mistake of wearing the wrong shape pants—wide on top and tapered at the bottom.) To bring out her eyes, we used black gel liner and smudged a deep plum powder shadow over it. Linda's skin was amazing, so she needed just a bit of tinted moisturizing balm and apricot blush to look her prettiest. For a more modern look, we swept her bangs to the side and blow-dried the ends straight to get rid of the flip.

Before "My style is very simple and casual. I use some bronzer, mascara, and a little bit of lip gloss. I usually blow-dry my hair and put in a few bobby pins when I go to sleep at night. I wear plain tops and pants; I hardly wear skirts and dresses anymore—I think it has to do with the fact that I've gained weight recently. I would love some help with my wardrobe."

After "I feel great about everything. I love the makeup and my hair. And more than anything, I'm amazed at how the clothes make me feel. The jeans make me look so much slimmer, and I realize that buying big clothes only makes me look bigger. I've learned some tricks to make my eyes pop more, and now I know how to define my eyebrows, which I've always felt look sparse in pictures."

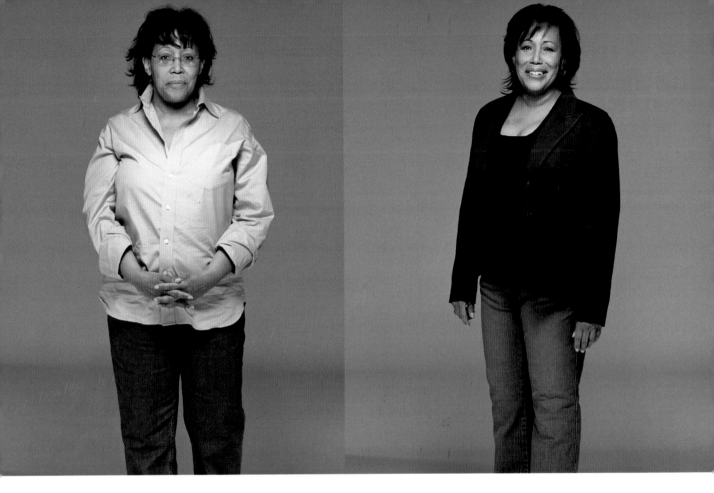

Linda's Tips You don't need to be slim to wear body-conscious clothes. I've always gone for large, boxy shapes and I'm now going to choose more fitted pieces.

Conditioner is important for relaxed hair. I've learned that I need to use a deep treatment at least twice a week (and I'll be mixing it with olive oil for added moisture).

Balance is key when it comes to makeup. If I go for a dramatic eye (by lining both upper and lower lash lines), I need to pair it with a nude lip color that looks like the color of my own lips.

A Life Changing Makeover
Suzanne Fee

What We Did Suzanne has taught all of my children. She is an amazing, bighearted woman, and one day I looked at Suzanne and knew that she could look so good if she just tweaked a few things. She is a beautiful woman, but her hair was overshadowing her looks. We covered the grays with a dark ash brown, tamed her hair by adding soft layers on top, then used a flatiron to straighten it. Suzanne had a lot of darkness under her eyes, so we used a combination of corrector and concealer to brighten up her face. Her lashes were a little sparse, so we created the illusion of more lashes by smudging dark powder shadow along her lash line (the black plum shade we chose brought out the green flecks in her eyes). To keep Suzanne's signature red lips from washing out the rest of her face, we warmed up her cheeks with a pale pink blush. Now she reminds me of a beautiful Italian opera star.

Before "I don't want to fuss too much. At this point in my life I'd rather read, walk the dog, or knit than spend time on my appearance. As far as makeup, I usually wear lipstick if nothing else. I've got a few gray hairs, but I haven't felt the need to color my hair because I feel like I've earned the grays. My hair is naturally curly and I tend to wear it like that, though I will occasionally blow-dry it to relax some of the curls. I'm basically happy with myself, but I don't usually feel like I look fantastic."

After "When I looked in the mirror, I saw myself in a whole new way. I felt gorgeous—like a queen. I realized that there's a really powerful connection between inner and outer beauty. Looking good makes you feel better about yourself...and when you feel better, it makes it easier to contemplate the other pieces in your life. After so many years of taking care of everyone around me, I'm just now starting to focus on myself. This makeover has given me a much-needed spark. At first I thought the new hair color was too dark, but I now think that it actually makes my complexion look better. And most of all, I love having my hair straight."

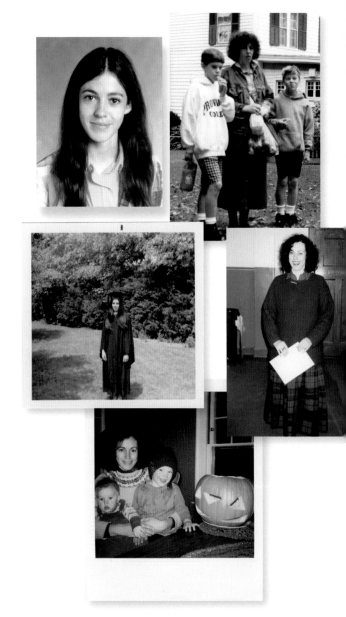

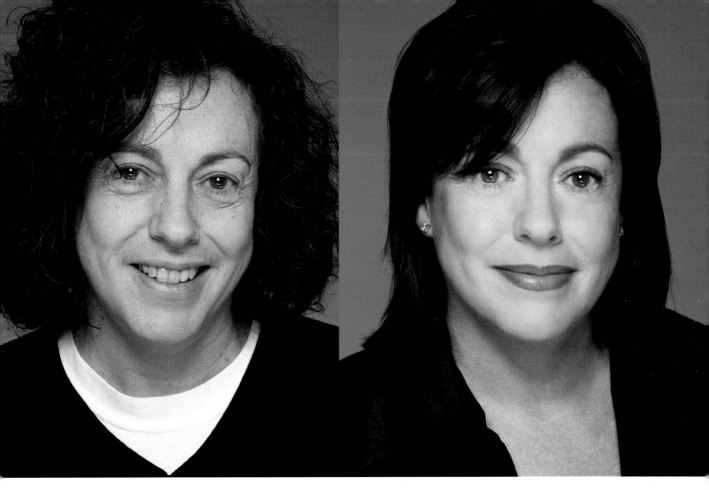

Suzanne's Tips Use a light hand (literally!) when you apply your makeup. I learned to pat, rather than rub, my under-eye concealer to blend it in.

If you have trouble managing your hair, ask your hairstylist for pointers. I've added a flatiron to my routine and it's made the biggest difference in how my hair looks.

To thine own self be true! Do and be what is right for you!

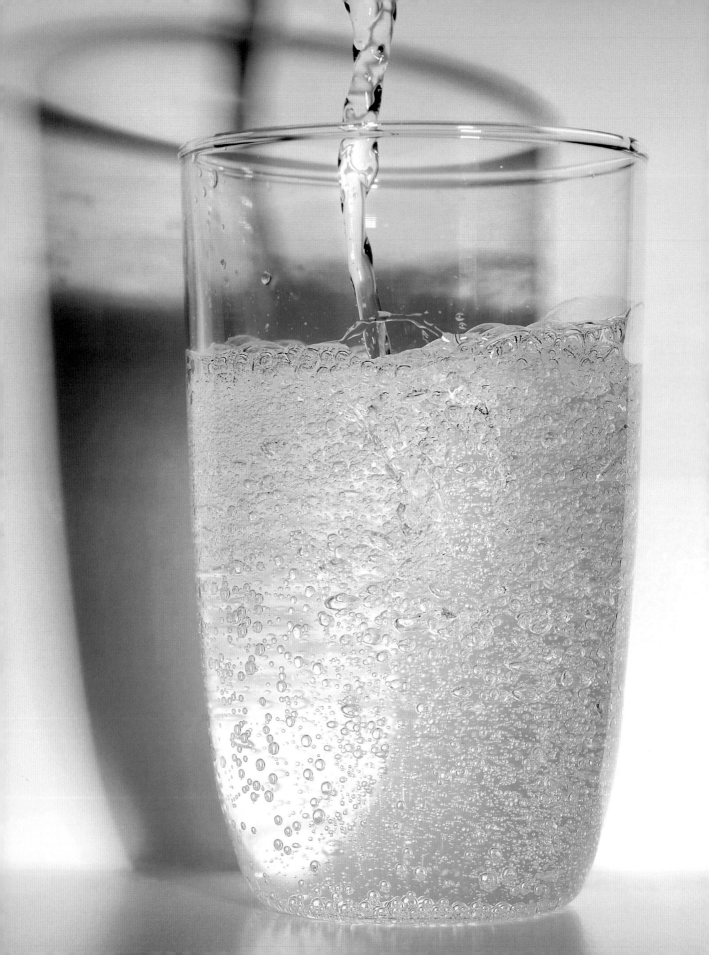

CHAPTER 9

BEAUTIFUL INSIDE & OUT

Women Who Get It

There are some women who always look great. It's not that they are more beautiful than other women. It's just that they know how to put it all together from head to toe. I can't help but stare—they look so pretty and seem so confident, and the best part is that they make it seem effortless. These women just "get it." But what is "it"? It's having an innate sense of style and being savvy in terms of fashion and beauty. The women featured in this chapter are great examples of what the rest of us aspire to, so I asked them to share their secrets for looking and feeling good.

Maureen Case
PRESIDENT, BOBBI BROWN COSMETICS

Beauty is confidence—in your bearing, the way you dress, the way you conduct yourself with others. It's about assurance. I believe that a positive outlook on life most affects the way you look. And the benefits of exercise and proper nutrition are undeniable; certainly they both require a lot of discipline, but the truism about "if you feel good, you will look good" is my guiding force. "Relentless optimism" has served me well.

As I get older, I deliberately focus on the good things in my life. Negativity about what you don't have does nothing to correct your situation. I find that an emphasis on what's right with the world usually has a ripple effect on those around me.

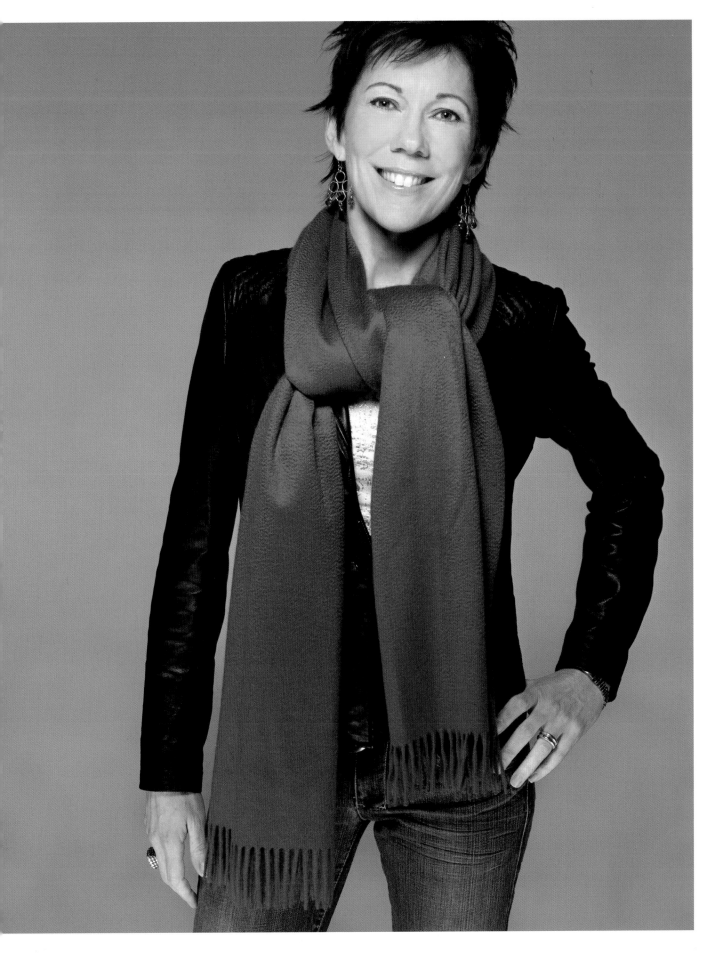

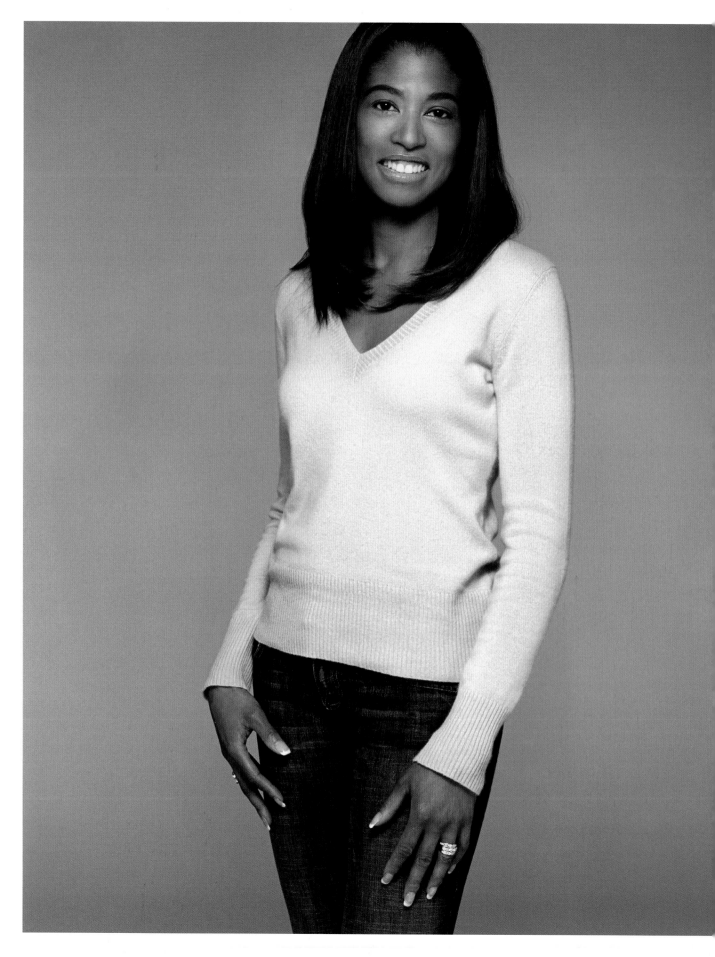

Terri Borden
FASHION CONSULTANT

I feel better in my forties than I ever have! I'm embracing my age as it goes on and I don't have any problem with aging as long as I work out and feel healthy. There's no better exercise than running after my kids. I've been taught that less is more when it comes to one's beauty regimen and I've adhered to this mantra all my life—I use cleanser, a simple moisturizer, and minimal makeup (lip gloss, a little eyeliner, and some bronzing powder).

Tiina Laakkonen
FASHION STYLIST

Beauty happens when you finally become friends with yourself and your features. It's about relaxing in your skin and being comfortable with the things that make you you. The great thing about getting older is that it's so much a state of mind and you can finally say, "OK, I don't look so bad." I've always been a firm believer in the adage that "less is more."

I care for my face with a simple regimen of water, moisturizer, and the occasional scrub. What you eat and how you live your life—these are the things that really show on your face.

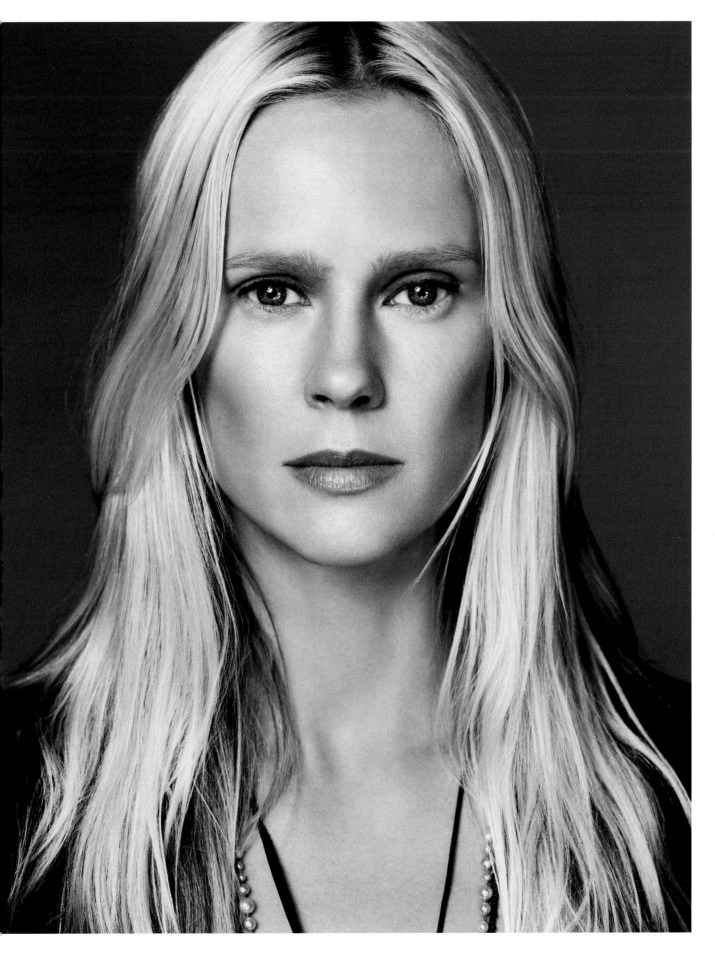

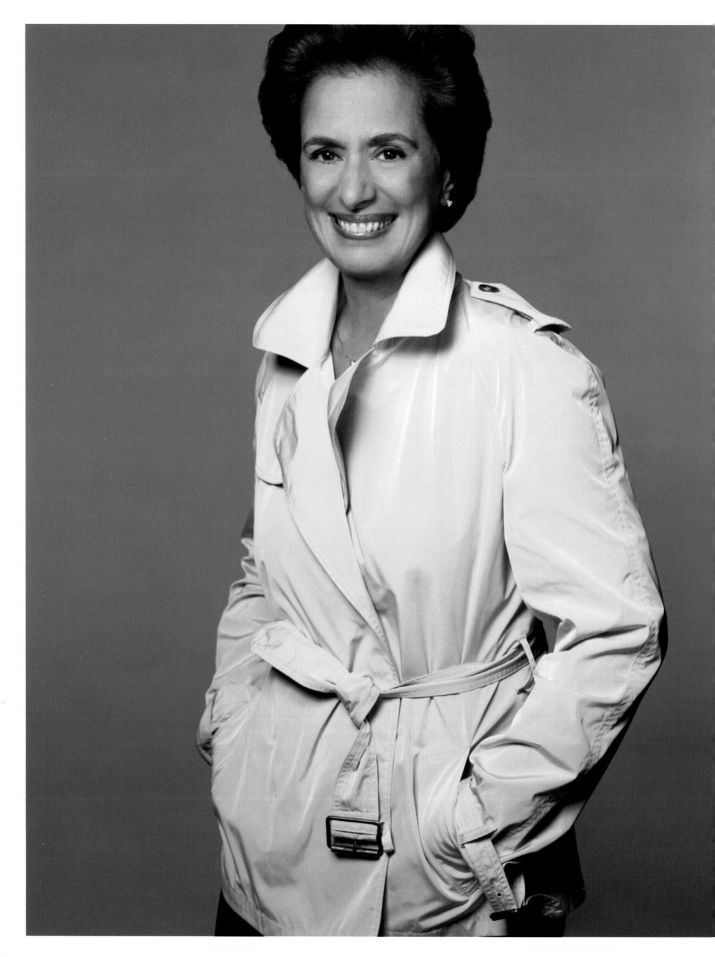

Rose Marie Bravo
VICE CHAIRMAN, BURBERRY

Beauty begins inside a human being and is about the spirit and soul of a person. This is a very precious and unique ingredient that determines each individual. Everybody is beautiful in his or her own way. Feeling good about yourself, your work, your family—that reflects in how you look. As I get older, I am dealing with the changes with the help of the Serenity Prayer..."accepting the things I cannot change, the courage to change the things that I can, and the wisdom to know the difference." Recognizing the changes as we age are warning lights telling us to enjoy the moment and cherish those we love.

Robin Brooks
CEO, BROOKS FOOD GROUP

My philosophy is that if you feel beautiful, you look beautiful. To accomplish that, I try to minimize any stress and start my day with exercise. A morning walk on the beach gives me a feeling of peace and serenity. I also work out with weights and practice yoga. I appreciate life and my surroundings.

I keep a well-hydrated, clean system. I keep my brows arched to frame my face and regularly dye my lashes and brows. I always have on hand a few necessary skincare and cosmetic products—for example, a good cleanser, misting water, moisturizer, eye cream, sun block of SPF 30 or higher, a sienna color stick for my cheeks, mascara, and lip gloss.

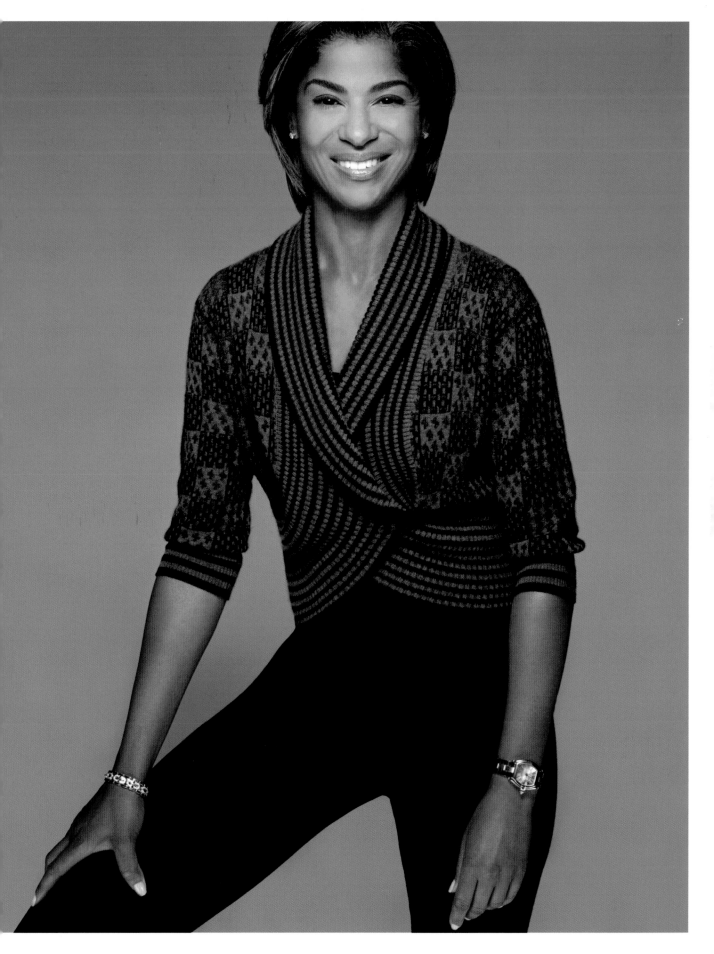

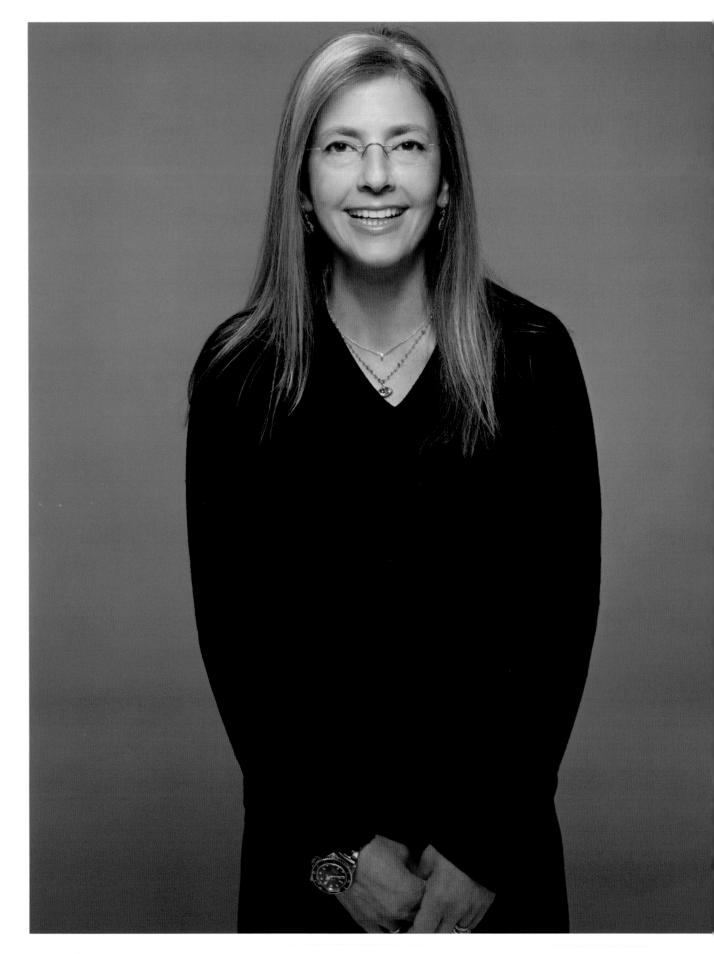

Ola Itani-Chan
VIP SERVICES/PERSONAL SHOPPER, PRADA BROADWAY

I believe in simplicity and natural beauty. Walking, swiming, meditation, and foot massages, combined with a healthy diet (vegetables, white meat, fish, red meat on occasion, and a glass of red wine) help me look and feel my best. I wash my face morning and night with cold water and face soap, and I always moisturize with face cream. I change my shampoo and conditioner once a month, and I'm careful with chamomile as it turns grey hair orange.

When it comes to fashion, my advice is to feel comfortable, beautiful, and a bit sexy in your garment. I believe in feeling young at heart, enjoying my grey hair, and embracing life day by day with a smile. I am grateful for what I have and who I am, and I find happiness in my family and friends. Being angry will not get you anywhere, it just ages you faster.

Kelly Klein
PHOTOGRAPHER

Beauty has to come from within. It's not about your face, eyes, skin, or how tall you are. You can't rely on your looks to feel beautiful because looks change over the years. Beauty is about your soul and your spirit. If you feel good about yourself as a person and you're happy being with yourself, then I think you're a complete, beautiful person. Beauty is waking up in the morning, opening your eyes, and feeling good without looking in the mirror.

I've always been very low maintenance. I don't do a lot for myself in terms of body treatments, facials, or creams and potions. But I always make sure to get a good night's rest. When the sun rises, I wake. And when the sun sets, I start to wind down. I think sleeping well is doing a lot to "preserve" me.

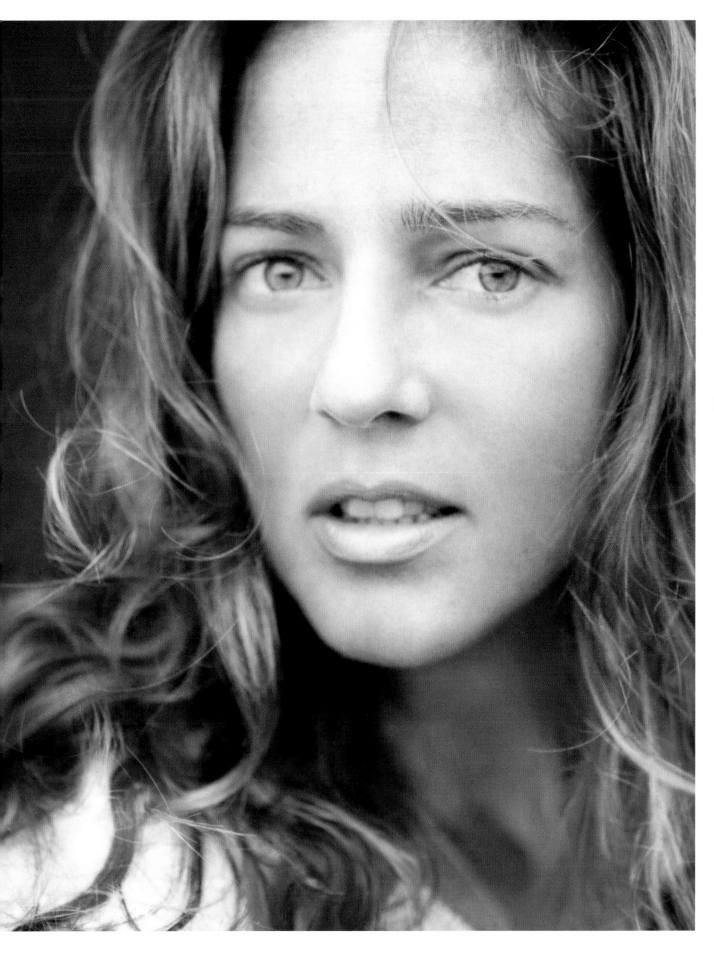

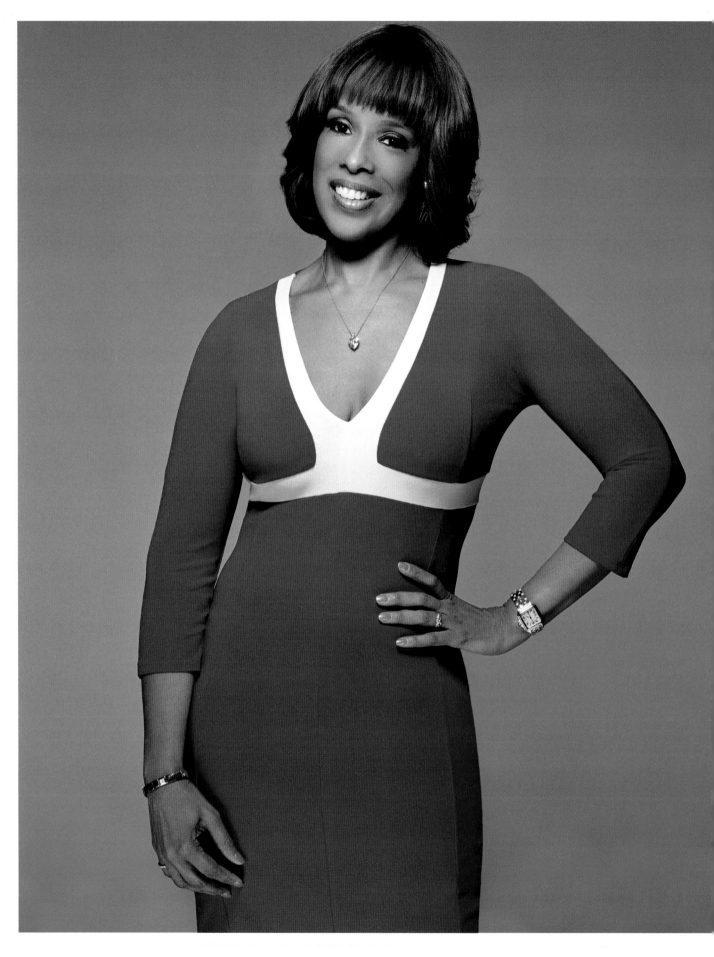

Gayle King
EDITOR AT LARGE, *O, THE OPRAH MAGAZINE*

My grandmother told me at age twenty-one, "Mother Nature wasn't as kind to you as she was to other little girls. You need to start wearing makeup." For years I believed that was true. While I swear by the talents of a good hair and makeup team, and utilize them often, I've also reached a time in my life that I so appreciate my natural face.

There's always going to be someone who people will consider more beautiful, but since I'm comfortable in my own skin, I feel pretty good all the time. And when all else fails, my favorite shade of lipstick can work wonders. I've discovered the value of strength training. In my case it has totally reshaped my body and makes my bones very happy. The older you get, the more important exercise becomes. Annoying, but oh so true. As it turns out, your mom was right—you should eat lots of vegetables and a little less cake.

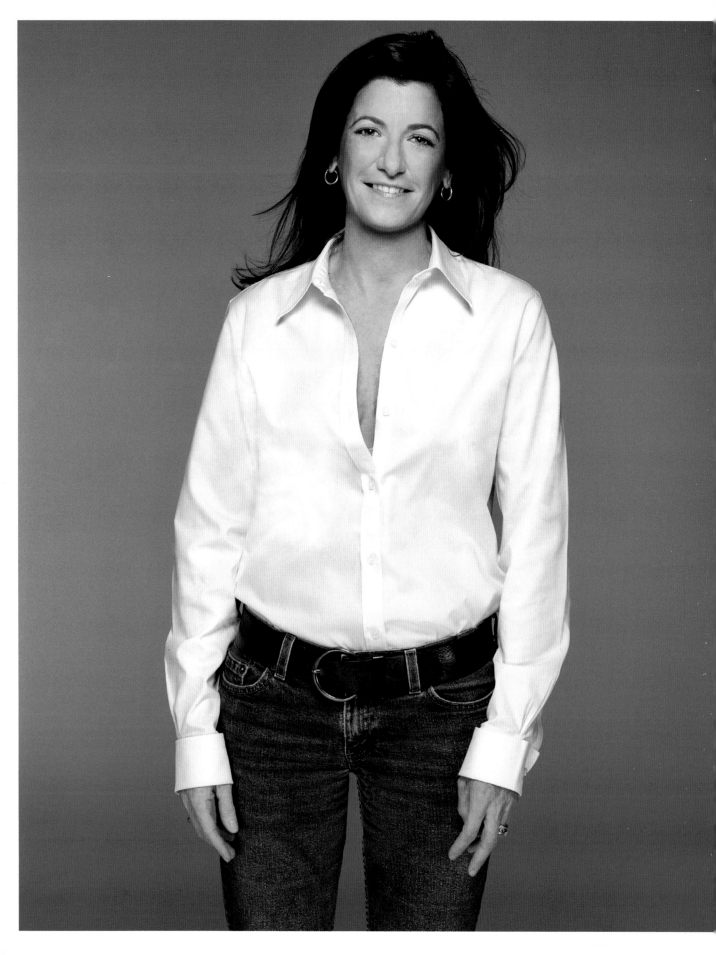

Jane Sarkin
FEATURES EDITOR, *VANITY FAIR*

My family is what gives me any kind of beauty that I have. When I see my children and my husband happy, that makes me happy. I think I look better now than when I was younger and I believe it has a lot to do with the fact that I have a very full life. In terms of beauty, I've always believed in keeping fuss to a minimum—one process for hair and just a cleanser and moisturizing cream for my face. Almost no makeup at all during the day, some when I go out. I love long hair and ponytails.

Time goes fast, so enjoy every minute as much as possible. Try to keep calm, stay healthy, eat as healthy as possible, and get as much sleep as you can. Think young.

Jill Cohen
NEW BUSINESS DEVELOPMENT, BOBBI BROWN COSMETICS

Beauty is about feeling comfortable and confident. Being fit and feeling healthy. Knowing how to take care of myself—both mind and body. All of those elements in balance create what I consider true beauty. Exercising every day has made a huge difference in my life. Once you start daily exercise you tend to eat carefully and choose healthier foods. I like the sun, but I never lay out anymore. Instead, I'll sit outside for fifteen minutes during a lunch break and soak in the sun. I've also learned that I feel best and most put together in simple, well-tailored clothing. At the end of the day, I feel most beautiful when I'm with my daughters, husband, and close friends having a great meal outside on a warm night.

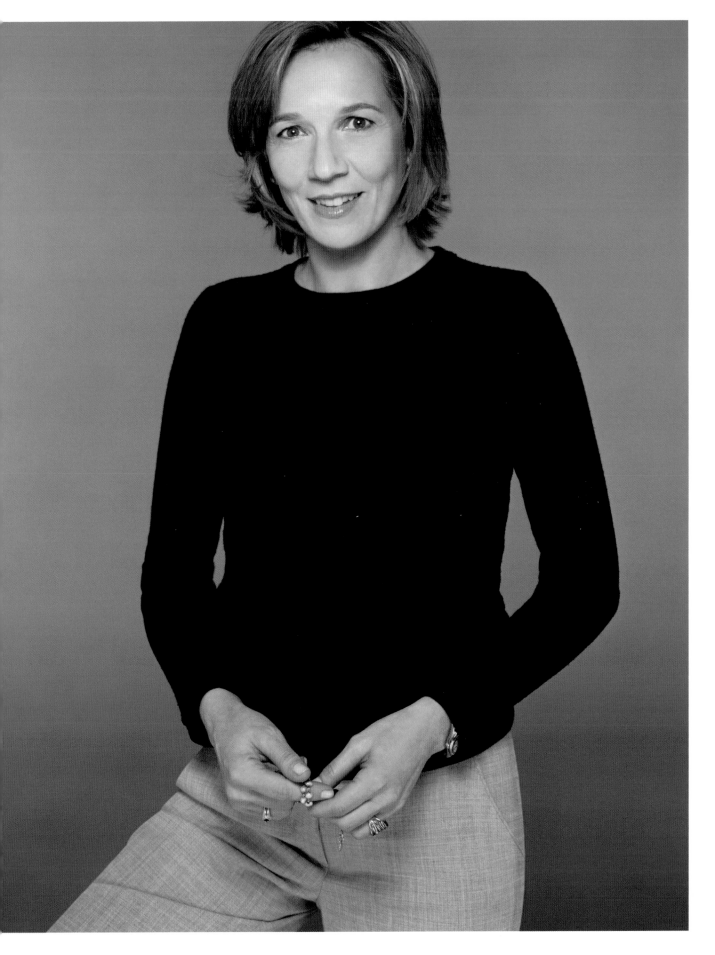

Lynn Tesoro
PARTNER, HL GROUP

I think I've always had a natural approach to beauty and it's become more apparent in recent years. I keep things simple and effortless. I feel comfortable doing what I want to do. I know what's "me" and I don't waste time focusing on things that are unachievable. I'm pretty religious about doing some kind of physical activity every day—whether it's running or my new passion, riding.

If I'm able to work out at the start of the day, I feel acomplished. Even if I've been out late the night before and feel awful, getting myself to the gym is the thing that allows me to function. I don't have any big secrets to looking good. I laugh a lot...in my opinion that's the best skin enhancer!

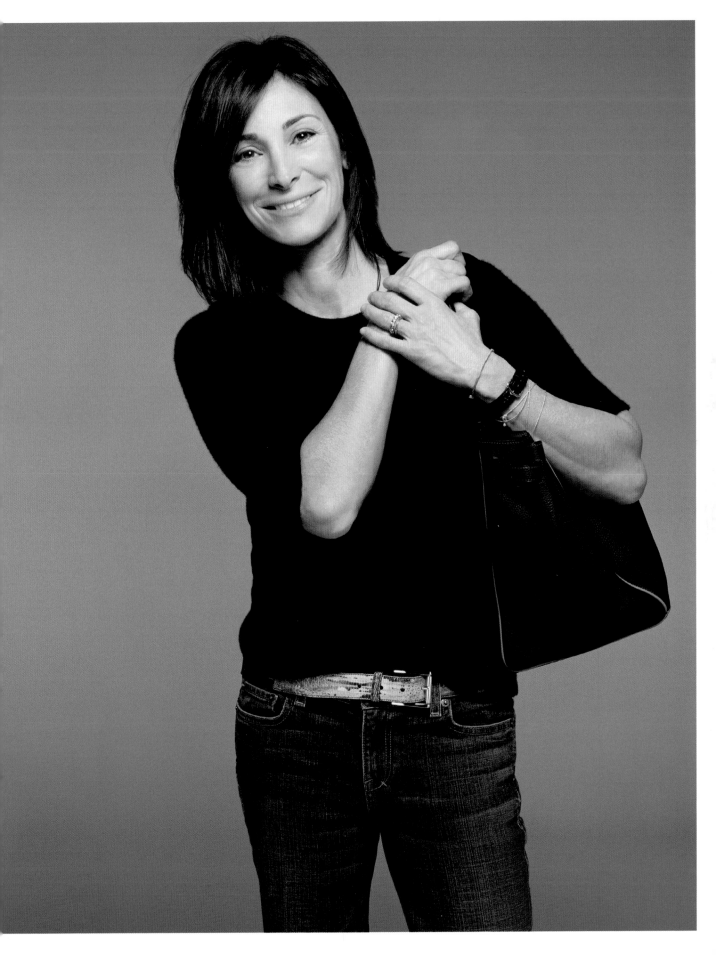

Conclusion
Create Your New Ideal

Living Beauty is a celebration of the journey that I, like many of my friends, am now embarking on. I've learned that it's not about looking young for your age—it's about looking great for your age. It's not about a number on the scale—it's about being strong. It's not about erasing the lines on your face—it's about achieving smooth skin. It's not about striving for perfection—it's about being really good. It's not about doing more—it's about learning to do less. And it's not about having more—it's about having better.

Having talked to my girlfriends and the countless women I work with, it's become really clear to me that it's those of us who are positive and open to growth who ultimately enjoy this journey. The women who are negative and afraid of what's to come are setting themselves up for only failure and disappointment, and I hope that this book will help turn things around for them.

Remember that your life is a big work in progress. Sometimes you have to take a few steps back in order to go forward. You'll experience many peaks and a fair share of valleys. When you find yourself in a negative place, the trick is to reevaluate your course and figure out what you need to do to get yourself back to a positive place. It's easy to feel bad, but I believe it's even easier to find something that will make you feel better. For me, it's eating healthy, exercising often, and always having a plan.

My plan is to continue to seek and be open to things that will allow me to grow and be a better person. I see endless possibilities ahead for myself and for the women of my generation, and I hope this book helps you create your own plan. This is what I've learned in my forty-ninth year:

- **Blaze, a Canyon Ranch fitness trainer, taught me that if it hurts, I shouldn't do it. Instead, I should do it a different way so it doesn't hurt.**

- **Watching Oprah Winfrey I've learned that stronger is the way to go.**

- **Yoga guru Jen Khol has shown me how to really plant my palms on the ground when I'm in down dog.**

- **From Jill Cohen I've learned that there is an invisible rubber band between my kids and me.**

- **Yogi Berra reminds me that you're never too old to cry.**

- **Leonard Lauder has taught me that you can never stop.**

- **My dad James Brown tells me to compartmentalize and do one thing at a time.**

- **Watching Adam Sandler in the movie *Click* I learned that we shouldn't wish away all those annoying tasks. It's called life and it goes fast enough anyway.**

- **And the best advice, from my husband Steven Plofker, "Breathe."**

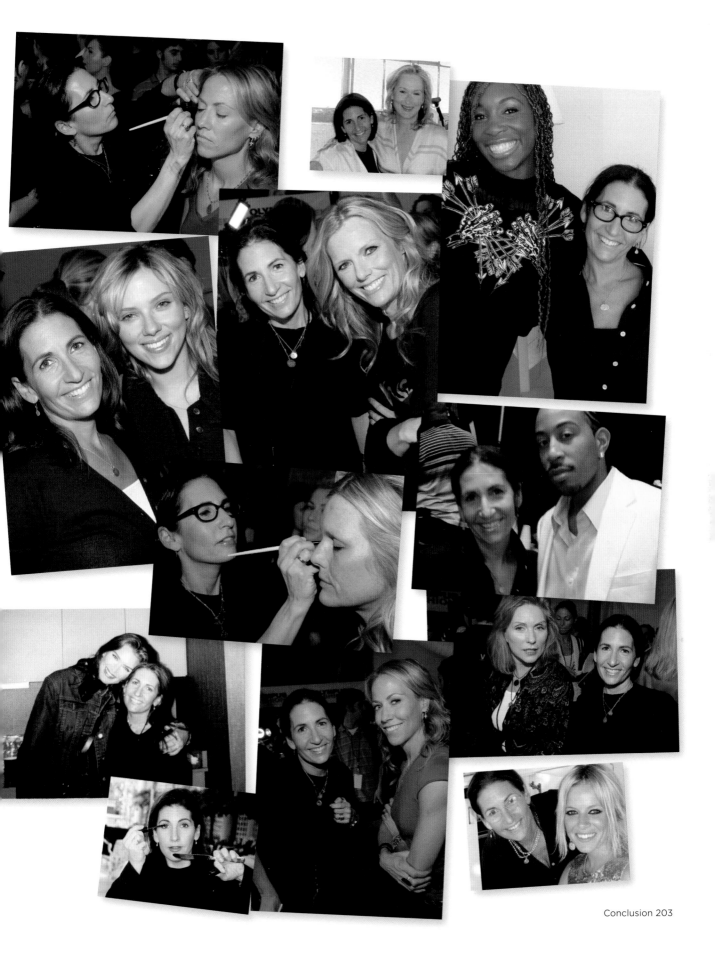

Acknowledgments

Special Acknowledgments

Ruba Abu-Nimah for your eyes and hands.

Amy Berkower for your foresight and stubbornness.

Maureen Case for your constant support and friendship.

Jill Cohen for your brain.

Marie Clare Katigbak-Sillick for your words and just being you.

Henry Leutwyler for your vision and humor.

Other Thanks

Models

Roshi Ameri
Nora Ariffin
Linda Arrandt
Joey Baffico
Linda Berkovic
Isisara Bey
Margie Bogdanow
Terri Borden
Lorraine Bracco
Rose Marie Bravo
Robin Brooks
Elizabeth Calderone
Phyliss Collins
Abby Cooperberg
Ann Curry
Ann D'Alessandro
Athie Daniskas
Carole Dlugasch
Elaine Douglas
Mary Dowd
Naomi Drewitz
Donna Edbril
Linda Fann
Suzanne Fee
Deborah Fitzgerald
Gayle Friscia
Shannon Gibbons
Nancy Golden
Karina Gomez
Janine Greene
Marcia Gay Harden
Andrea Herbert
Susan Hersch
Ola Itani-Chan
Julie Jackson
Patricia Kimble
Gayle King
Kelly Klein
Tiina Laakkonen
Leslie Larson
Amy Lazarus
Gunilla Linblad
Deborah Loeffler
Colleen Maloney
Dorothy Mancuso
Rita Mangan
Sara Moss
Deborah Philips
Michelle Pinkalla
Bryna Plofker
Rose Rampersaud
Amy Rosen
Alix Ross
Karen Ross
Margita Rudovic
Ruby Sampson
Susan Sarandon
Jane Sarkin
Susan Saunders
Marva Smalls
Sharon Sodikoff
Mary Steenburgen
Nancy Sturino
Lynn Tesoro
Fatim Thiam
Lisa Travis
Marie Rose Tricon
Sharon Burton Turner
Jaime Walter
Vera Wang

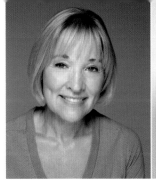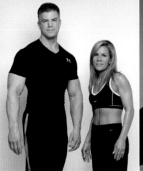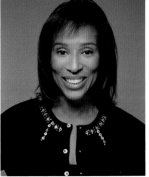

Barb Westfield
Quintell Williams
Vanessa Williams
Rita Wilson
Debra Winger

Experts
Anna Chiommino
Dr. Gerald Ciciola
Dr. Kenneth Y. Davis
Dr. Jeanine B. Downie
Dr. Christiane Northrup
Dr. Joseph Raffaele
Dr. Jairo Rodriguez
Chris Edwards at BriteSmile
Rich Fitter at Platinum
  Fitness
Molly Fox
Deborah Furr at Johari
Camilla Huey
Lori Kaplan
Marcia Kilgore at Bliss Spa
David Kirsch at Madison
  Square Club
Sarah Robbins
Monica Trentin at
  Platinum Fitness

Makeup
Loran Alvator
Katrina Danson
Ricki Gurtman
Gregg Hubbard
Ellice Schwab
Kimberly Soane
Sebastien Tardif
Cynde Watson-Richmond

Hair
Mario Diab
Genevieve Enriquez
Julie McIntosh
Alexandra Taralesca

Styling
Kristen Boscaino
Deborah Medeiros-Baker

Wardrobe
7 For All Mankind
Bra*Tenders
Chantelle
Diana Heimann
Lauren Harper Collection
Lord & Taylor
Only Hearts
Pure Color Jeans
Sassybax
SPANX
Theory
Wacoal

Photography
John Cassidy
Matthias Gaggl
Daymion Mardel
Jason Nakleh

Marketing & Publicity
Ashley Badger-Wakefield
Matthew Ballast
Gretchen Berra
Candice Burd
Courtney Mulligan
Veronika Ullmer

Special Services
Chris Berry
John Eaton
Ron Hill
Michelle Howry
Hirut Selek Kebede (Ruth)
Al Lewis
Raven McGrath
Karen Murgolo
David Nass
Jamie Raab
Jodi Reamer
Craig Rose
Charlotte Rowe
Katie Sturino
Hermes Zambrano

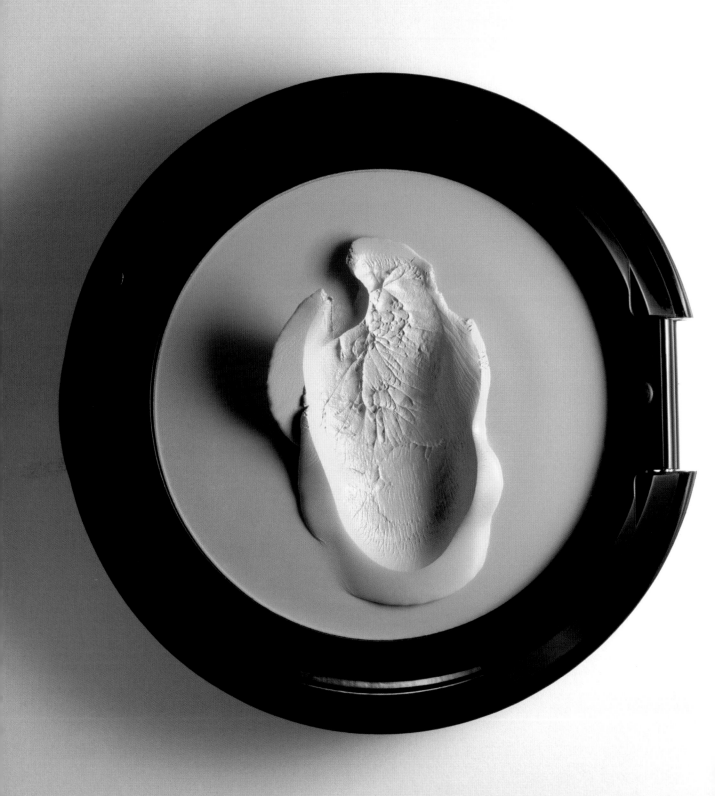